A Manual of
Interpersonal Skills for Nurses:
An experiential approach

A MANUAL OF INTERPERSONAL SKILLS FOR NURSES:
An experiential approach

Carolyn Kagan,
Lecturer in Social Psychology,
Manchester Polytechnic

Josie Evans,
Lecturer in Health Studies,
Lancashire Polytechnic

Betty Kay,
Senior Tutor, Salford School of Nursing

Harper & Row, Publishers
London

Philadelphia
New York
St. Louis
Sydney

San Francisco
London
Singapore
Tokyo

First published 1986, 1987
Reprinted 1989

Harper & Row Ltd
28 Tavistock Street
London WC2E 7PN

British Library Cataloguing in Publication Data
Kagan, Carolyn
   A manual of interpersonal skills for nurses: an experiential approach.
   1.   Nurse and patient
   I.   Title
   610.73′06′99   RT86
   ISBN 0-6-318356-0

Typeset by Burns and Smith Ltd, Derby
Printed and bound by The Alden Press, Oxford

For our students

CONTENTS

PREFACE

We believe it is important for you to know something about how this book has been written if you, as reader, are to be able to put what you find here in some perspective. It has been written collaboratively. Carolyn Kagan wrote the first draft and devised initial versions of all the exercises. Josie Evans and Betty Kay read, commented, altered and added to these drafts, creating substantial changes. We all discussed the changes and have experimented with the exercises. The whole process has taken two years. This is a long time but did not seem long at all as we tried to refine the material in response to student comment and experience. The process of modification will continue, and we hope that you will feel confident to make your own changes in the light of your own experience with the material. What we hope we are offering here are some ideas and activities that we, and our students, have been able to work with constructively. It is often difficult to identify the source of structured exercises and activities in the development of helping skills. We think we have arrived at our own adaptations of familiar and unfamiliar exercises. If, however, any reader feels that we should have credited her/him with an original idea, and that we have failed to do this, we apologize.

We have all been involved with interpersonal skills teaching and learning with a variety of nursing students for about nine years. Carolyn came from a background in social psychology: her research and teaching interests have been in the fields of interpersonal behaviour, social skills training and the development of helping relationships. She is not a nurse, but is indebted to the nursing staff she met as a consumer between 1974 and 1984 from the following nursing settings: Nuffield Orthopaedic Hospital, Oxford;

Manchester Royal Infirmary; Park Hospital, Davyhulme; Withington Hospital, Manchester; Trafford and South Manchester Community Nursing Services; Stretford Memorial Hospital. Many of her observations of nurse–patient interactions are contained in this book. Carolyn has also learnt a lot from students of various nursing courses at Manchester Polytechnic since 1976, and from the staff in the nursing section who have offered support and encouragement in the development of interpersonal skills work on their courses, before the area of work was given unequivocal support from the professional validating bodies.

Josie has a nursing background, having undertaken basic general and district nurse training with Salford Health Authority. Following wide and varied experience in different nursing areas, she has been involved in basic and post-basic nurse education for approximately eight years. Her particular clinical interests lie in intensive care/coronary care nursing and in terminal care. Research and teaching interests mirror both this clinical involvement and a strong commitment to the development of communication skills training in professional nursing.

Betty undertook her general nurse training at Manchester Royal Infirmary and trained as a health visitor at Manchester Polytechnic. She worked as a nurse tutor at Park Hospital, Davyhulme, before obtaining her present post as a senior tutor at the Salford School of Nursing, where she has worked for the past nine years. She developed an interest in the teaching of interpersonal skills to nursing students after undertaking the BSc in nursing studies at Manchester Polytechnic. She is indebted to the student nurses who have cooperated in the interpersonal skills sessions.

Our teaching and writing takes up only part of our lives. We all have families who have borne our preoccupation during the last two years. Carolyn has young children and would like to offer thanks to Helen Mortimer, whose imaginative work with them has helped them understand why their mother must work in the evenings and at weekends and is constantly tired! Mark Burton has helped Carolyn turn her observations and teaching experiences into a form that can be shared, by enthusiastically taking responsibility for domestic affairs and child care, and by discussing her work with her endlessly, thus helping her focus her ideas. Other friends have waited patiently for a time that she is not engrossed in her book. She would like to thank them all.

Josie would like to thank her immediate family, particularly her husband Gerald, for their constant support, practical help and encouragement during the last few years. Also, grateful thanks are extended to her (now grown-up) children, David, Lisa and Gareth for coping so well and patiently whilst their 'absent' Mum was working. In addition, thanks to Chris, Dorothea and friends who listened so effectively. Josie also much appreciates the encouragement, staunch support and practical help offered by nursing/teaching colleagues at Salford and Preston.

Manuscripts do not prepare themselves. Carolyn has done a lot of the typing herself. However, thanks are also due to Mrs Meehan and the women in the Faculty Typing Unit at the Polytechnic, and to Janet Icely and Alison White for corrections of drafts. Ian Reid did some of the artwork. Our thanks go to all of them for their attempts to provide an efficient service in an institution that does little to support or encourage the writing of books. The staff at Harper and Row have been valuable sources of encouragement. Cathy Peck was an enthusiastic commissioning editor, and Griselda Campbell has had the arduous task of refining the final product. We appreciate the friendly support and patience that has been offered by them both.

Carolyn Kagan
Josie Evans
Betty Kay
Manchester January 1986

INTRODUCTION

The nature of interpersonal skill

Interpersonal skills refer to those interpersonal aspects of communication and social skills that people (need to) use in direct person-to-person contact. Not all communication is interpersonal: messages may be transmitted through any medium and may include televised, pictorial, written or tape-recorded messages. Similarly, not all social skills are interpersonal. In the health field social skill is taken to include those skills required to lead ordinary lives and may include how to eat 'properly' and how to use public transport or other community resources. For further discussion of both communication and social skills in nursing, see Bridge and MacLeod Clark (1981); Faulkner (1984); French (1983); Smith and Bass (1982).

To behave skilfully is to respond flexibly to changing circumstances in the pursuit of clear goals with maximum efficiency. Given this broad definition, several assumptions underlie a skills approach to interpersonal behaviour:

(a) There are cognitive (perceptual and interpretative) aspects of interpersonal behaviour as well as performance aspects.
(b) Interpersonal behaviours are learnt. It follows from this that they can be mislearnt (distorted), not learnt (absent) or better learnt (developed).
(c) Interpersonal behaviour can be broken down into components, each of which can be identified, practised and combined with others to improve overall levels of competence.

Interpersonal skills training has been devised for many different 'student' groups. The focus has tended to be on those people with interaction 'problems' such as psychologically disabled people (Trower *et al.*, 1978) and delinquent children and adolescents (Priestley *et al.*, 1979; Spence, 1982) as well as those from different professional groups, including nurses (Sidney *et al.*, 1973; Ellis and Whittington, 1981). Training programmes have varied with the need of the student groups and are currently incorporating important conceptual and methodological issues that have emerged from an expanding field (Ellis and Whittington, 1983; Spence and Shepherd, 1983; Trower, 1984).

Interpersonal skills and nursing

Nursing is an interpersonal activity in so far as most of the things that nurses do involve at least one other person. To do their job nurses bring the interpersonal skills that work for them in their everyday lives and apply them at work. But something happens when they do this. Time and time again, research into the effectiveness of nurses' communication and interpersonal skills has shown them to be sadly lacking. Even taking into account that hospitals (and other health care settings) are strange and unique places where strange things happen to people, it seems that nurses readily succumb to external and internal pressures to discard and distort their interpersonal skills (see Faulkner [1984] and Kagan [1985] for some recent reviews of this literature). There are some specialist interpersonal skills (such as assessment, giving appropriate information, assertiveness, counselling, etc.) that nurses may not have had the chance to learn previously, and some settings (such as intensive care) that are totally alien to them. In these cases it is hardly surprising that they fail to use appropriate skills. However, the bulk of nurses' time is spent in more informal interaction with patients, relatives and colleagues, and here nurses seem to fare rather better. Nevertheless, researchers in the field make persistent pleas for interpersonal skills to be included in basic and post-basic nurse education. Furthermore, with the incorporation of the 'nursing process' and individualized patient care into many nursing settings, professional validating bodies are beginning to express their concern over nurses' ineffective use of interpersonal skills, a concern that is emerging in syllabus guidelines. Thus there is considerable pressure to teach interpersonal skills to nurses.

We would argue that there are several levels at which interpersonal skills teaching should be directed. Firstly, nurses need to *develop insight* into their own interpersonal skills in order to recognize why they may not be using them effectively in their work settings. It is only with this recognition that they might be able to overcome some of the barriers — both internal and external — that they meet. Secondly, (some) nurses need to *learn specialist skills* and/or ways of extending skills to special settings. Thirdly, nurses must begin to know when and why to *use particular interpersonal strategies* and how to manage the effects they have. Fourthly, nurses need to explore some of the *constraints* that limit the effective use of interpersonal skills in clinical settings.

We see, then, the teaching/learning of interpersonal skills as a process which goes on and on, rather than as a body of knowledge that can be taught/learnt once and for all. Nurses will always be able to improve their interpersonal skills, however 'good' they are at the moment. It is the insight into, evaluation and ability to change their own interpersonal behaviour that will enable nurses to respond flexibly to changing circumstances in order to achieve their goals with responsiveness and maximum efficiency. These are the qualities of people who are interpersonally skilled.

This book aims to consider all three levels of interpersonal skill. The assumptions we make are clear:

(a) The use of effective interpersonal skill is a continuing process, not an end point.
(b) Self-awareness and insight into our own interpersonal functioning enable us to become interpersonally effective.
(c) Some specialist interpersonal skills can be identified and taught.
(d) The understanding, evaluation and change of interpersonal strategies is fundamental to interpersonal skill.
(e) Interpersonal skills take place in a social context which may inhibit their effective use.

A model of interpersonal skill

One of the major difficulties faced in organizing the material for this book was the lack of a simple model of interpersonal skills that included some of the complexities of nursing ·interactions as well as both theoretical and practical issues. There is no clear statement of what, exactly, the interpersonal skills needed by nurses are, although some writers have pointed in certain directions (see e.g. Kagan, 1985). Figure I is a heuristic device that we have

Figure I   A model of interpersonal skill

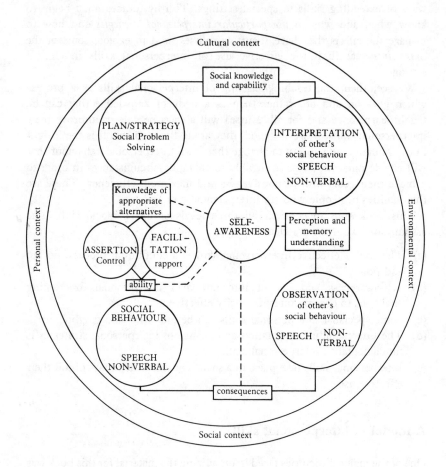

found useful in providing an overall conceptualization of interpersonal skills from which discrete teaching/learning modules may be selected: it is not meant to be a model of how interpersonal relations occur.

The chapters in this book reflect for the most part the modules in Figure I. Each module (and each chapter) has a discrete theoretical background and set of practical skills. Whichever 'module' is under consideration, self-awareness is seen to be central (sic) and the constraints proposed by different features of the nursing context must be taken into account. The different modules will be more or less important for different groups of students at different times, and it is not to be assumed that they are equally weighted.

How to use this book

Student groups have different needs in terms of interpersonal skills training, depending on their level of training, existing interpersonal skills, nursing specialisms, assessment requirements, and so on. Different courses have different amounts of time to spend on interpersonal skills training, and so tutors may want to be more or less selective in what they cover. We hope that although each chapter could be treated as a discrete unit, all the chapters are presented in a coherent sequence, should readers wish to integrate the topics.

The book can be used by individual people who wish to explore and develop their interpersonal skills on their own, by groups of interested people, or by tutors teaching interpersonal skills to classes of students.

We have discussed the theoretical background to a topic with examples from the nursing field. All the anecdotes and illustrations are drawn from real nursing situations: they really happened, although at times they may seem incredible. We have interspersed exercises and issues for reflection/discussion throughout the text, as we believe practising and experiencing to be the most effective way both to learn the implications of what is being suggested and to keep the theoretical discussion firmly rooted in a practical context. We see no virtue in debating theory that has little practical use, nor of practising skills in the isolation of theoretical background. In the text we have omitted detailed references, but all the comment is based on research findings from social psychology, sociology and nursing fields. The reading supplied at the end of each chapter should lead the critical reader to relevant material.

We would hope that any tutors conducting interpersonal skills classes would have had some appropriate training. However, the reality is that many will not have had any. Interpersonal skills will be taught by people with little experience (and perhaps little interest) in the field. We have, therefore, included a section on notes for tutors who wish to use the exercises in class (Appendix I). We hope the notes help the sessions to run smoothly, although they cannot cover every eventuality. Tutors must be prepared to deal with the unexpected in class and to experience heights of satisfaction and depths of frustration as groups of students respond differently to similar course material. This will be inevitable as students bring a variety of experiences, attitudes, values and opinions to bear on interpersonal skills work. It is this, perhaps more than anything, that makes interpersonal skills teaching an exciting and rewarding field to work in. If this book contributes to that excitement for both tutors and students, it will have succeeded.

References

Bridge, W. and Macleod Clark, J. (Eds.) (1981) *Communication in Nursing Care,* H.M. and M. (Wiley), Aylesbury

Ellis, R.A.F. and Whittington, D. (1981) *A Guide to Social Skill Training,* Croom Helm, London

Ellis, R.A.F. and Whittington, D. (1983) *New Directions in Social Skill Training,* Croom Helm, London

Faulkner, A. (Ed.) (1984) *Recent Advances in Nursing, 7, Communication,* Churchill Livingstone, Edinburgh

French, P. (1983) *Social Skills and Nursing Practice,* Croom Helm, London

Kagan, C. (Ed.) (1985) *Interpersonal Skills in Nursing: Research and Applications,* Croom Helm, London

Priestley, P., McGuire, J., Flegg, D., Hemsley, V. and Welham, D. (1979) *Social Skills and Personal Problem Solving: a handbook of methods,* Tavistock, London

Sidney, E., Brown, M. and Argyle, M. (1973) *Skills with People,* Hutchinson, London

Smith, V.N. and Bass, T.A. (1982) *Communication in the Health Care Team,* Harper and Row, London

Spence, S. (1982) *Social Skills Training with Children and Adolescents: a practical manual,* NFER, London

Spence, S. and Shepherd, G. (1983) *Developments in Social Skills Training,* Academic Press, London

Trower, P. (Ed.) (1984) *Radical Perspectives in Social Skills Training,* Croom Helm, London

Trower, P., Bryant, B. and Argyle, M. (1978) *Social Skills and Mental Health,* Methuen, London

CHAPTER 1

TEACHING INTERPERSONAL SKILLS TO NURSES

Teaching and learning interpersonal skills is an exciting, often frustrating venture. There is no generally accepted content area nor any clear theoretical material that must be included. Instead the courses depend on the student group, time, and resources (including tutors) available.

1.1 Planning the course

Before starting an interpersonal skills course, careful consideration should be given to issues of resources, content, methods, structure, validity, tutors and students, as depicted in Figure 1.1

Tutors

Sometimes tutors will be teaching interpersonal skills because they want to, and they think the area important. Frequently though, tutors with no interest in the field may well find themselves being asked to teach it. Thus there is likely to be diversity in tutor motivation, as well as in their knowledge or experience of interpersonal skills work. Certain tutor qualities are essential for effective interpersonal skills teaching. The nature of the work requires tutors

Figure 1.1   Questions to ask at the start of interpersonal skills training

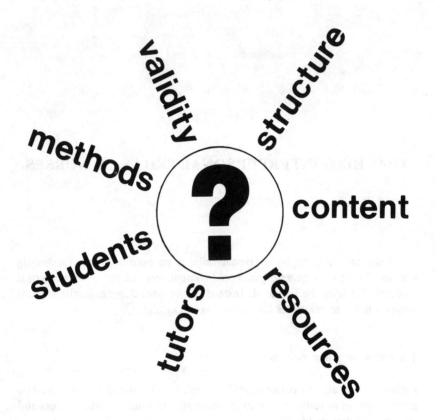

to be open and non-defensive, to be able to handle conflict (and perhaps distress) in the classroom and to have explored issues relating to their own levels of self-awareness. Tutors who have not developed these qualities may well find the teaching unrewarding or even stressful. We would urge that tutors entering the field for the first time do all they can to become involved in some experiential learning prior to starting their own courses. Tutors' own level of interpersonal skills will, too, affect the efficacy of their teaching.

Resources

Tutor resources are of critical importance to successful interpersonal skills training. So, too, are physical resources. The amount of time available, the suitability of classroom facilities (interpersonal skills work is often noisy and requires comfortable, relaxed surroundings), access to hardware such as video/audio tape equipment and library stocks, and the size of classes (12–15 students is optimal) will all influence the quality of the teaching/learning.

Because interpersonal skills teaching/learning can touch on personally sensitive areas, adequate provision for both tutor and student support should be available. Tutors may have to ensure that they are readily available for students to discuss any issues of personal concern.

Content

Decisions will have to made regarding the breadth and depth of coverage on a particular course. Criteria for including material will be linked to both tutor/student experience, resource issues and professional requirements. The links with other teaching areas and with the clinical field will need to be considered. It is often extremely useful to involve colleagues from other areas and from the clinical field in the planning of the interpersonal skills courses, both in order to enlist their cooperation and to ensure the practical utility of the material to be covered. Assessment requirements may, to a certain extent, influence the content of a course, but care should be taken to avoid a situation of 'the tail wagging the dog'.

Methods

By and large, interpersonal skills teaching will use experiential methods (see Section 1.2). There are several implications of this. Tutors must ensure that the planning of courses leaves plenty of time for students to practise the skills they learn, and for them to receive feedback on, and to process, their experiences. It is also necessary to allow time for tutors to prepare material carefully, as structured learning can be unproductive if poorly prepared. Some provision, too, should be made for monitoring and evaluating students' learning and teaching methods, etc., and for appropriate modifications to be made to courses.

Structure

As with all other curricula, careful consideration will need to be given to matters of organization within the course and to how the different elements fit in with students' other learning experiences. The links, too, with practical nursing will need to be clarified, and if feasible, clinical staff coopted onto the planning team. Individual sessions need careful training to allow space for consolidation and discussion, and some thought should be given to how students' homework and other experiences should be integrated in the classroom. Interpersonal skills teaching cannot take place in isolation from the rest of the students' lives.

Validity

The decisions that are made in the light of the issues raised above will affect the validity of the interpersonal skills courses. Tutors will need to consider the extent to which the course meets student and professional needs, whether appropriate assessment and evaluation methods can be devised (see Section 1.3) and what the connections between self-awareness, interpersonal understanding and skilled performance might be. Consideration of how the generalization of skill from one situation to another should be addressed, in conjunction with how the different facets of interpersonal skills mesh with each other, will be required.

Students

Students vary in terms of their existing levels of interpersonal skills, their attitudes and motivation and their degree of self-confidence/consciousness. These factors should be taken into account when planning and running interpersonal skills courses, as well as the composition of class groups in terms of similarities and dissimilarities between class members. Students will all have different expectations of an interpersonal skills course, and every effort should be made to ascertain these prior to, and during, individual courses.

Table 1.1 summarizes the issues that need to be considered before mounting an interpersonal skills course. This list is not an exhaustive one and there may well be some more that we should have included. The message, though, is clear: *interpersonal skills courses require careful and extensive preparation and should be modified according to resources, student needs and tutor expertise.*

1.2 Experiential learning

In this book, we have adopted, along with other workers in the field, an experiential approach to interpersonal skills learning and teaching. This means that students are asked to carry out a variety of practical tasks that will enable them directly to experience the subject matter for themselves. There are many different ways that experiential learning can be brought about (see Tomlinson [1985] for a review). We have used, in the main, structured exercises, whereby students are given tasks to do and then to discuss in the light of specific issues, linking their experiences to both the theoretical and work contexts. If the exercises are used in classroom settings, tutors have a facilitative rather than participative role: in other words their task is to create the conditions whereby students can derive maximum benefit from the exercises. At times this may require tutors to become involved with groups if they get 'stuck', but at other times to remain as unobtrusive as possible whilst ensuring that students engage in appropriate activity. No tutor should, however, ask students to do anything that she/he has not done her/himself — or at least would not be prepared to do. Tutors have responsibility to create a safe working environment for students and this will require them to be open and non-defensive about themselves and their teaching. For many tutors this will not be easy, but reluctance (or inability) to do so will detract from the value of the interpersonal skill sessions.

Table 1.1   Issues to consider before starting interpersonal skills training

Tutors	Resources	Content	Methods
Who?	Time	Breadth and depth of coverage	Implications of experiential methods
Motivation	Personal and technical support	Inclusion criteria	Sensitization
Knowledge and experience	Location and suitability of accommodation	Links with theory	Opportunities to practise
Openness and non-defensiveness	Number of staff	Links with other areas	Feedback and processing
Self-awareness	Availability hardware (video/audio facilities)	Links with clinical field	Preparation and provision of materials
Ability to handle conflict	Availability teaching aids	Links with professional bodies	Monitoring and evaluation
Levels of IPS	Access to well-stocked library	Assessment	
	Class size		

Structure	Validity	Students	Others?
Overall course links with other areas	Assessment criteria	Level IPS	
Links with practical nursing	Monitoring and change	Attitudes and motivation	
Individual sessions	Links with clinical field	Self-confidence	
Integration of homework and experience	Self-awareness	Self-consciousness	
	Interpersonal knowledge	Class composition (similarity/differences with others)	
		Anxiety	

Learning contract

Students, too, have responsibilities with regard to experiential learning. If they are using this book by themselves they should undertake to give serious consideration to the discussion issues relating to the exercises, preferably by talking with colleagues about them. In classroom settings students have responsibilities to each other to carry out the tasks set, including homework tasks, and to give due consideration to the implications of their experiences. Experiential learning will be of optimum value if students participate fully and honestly. One way to encourage students to accept responsibility for participating in an experiential learning course is to negotiate a 'learning contract' with them at the start. An example of a learning contract is shown in Figure 1.2

Progress and change

Interpersonal skills learning, as we have argued before, is a process and not an outcome. It is not going to be a case of 'now I don't have interpersonal skill ... now I have interpersonal skill', so students can sometimes feel as if they are not learning anything new. It is, therefore, a good idea to include some methods whereby students can monitor their own progress and change. It is often helpful to invite students to think about their expectations of an interpersonal skills course, right at the beginning of the course, and if possible to identify some of their own learning goals. An 'expectations and goals' schedule is presented in Exercise 1.1

Students should not be expected to have sophisticated insight into their own interpersonal behaviour, but rather to think around what interpersonal skills in nursing means to them. These expectations and goals are personal ones and need not form the basis of class discussion; if the exercise is repeated at intervals throughout training, a valuable record of change can be made. One way in which tutors can start to create an open teaching atmosphere is by completing Exercise 1.1 themselves in relation to the course and sharing their hopes with the students.

Figure 1.2   A learning contract

I understand that I will be taking an experiential approach to learning about the nature of interpersonal relationships and to develop the skills needed to function effectively as a nurse. I understand that there will be some theoretical input to the course and that there will be assessments at the end of each unit.

I willingly accept the following statements:

1. I will use the structured experiences in the course to learn from. This means I am willing to engage in specified behaviours, seek out feedback and analyze my interpersonal interactions with other class members in order to make the most of my learning.

2. I will make the most of my own learning by:
   (a) engaging in specified activities and in being open about my feelings and reactions to what is taking place;
   (b) setting my own goals that I will work actively to accomplish — which means that I will take responsibility for my own learning and not wait around for someone else to teach me;
   (c) being willing to experiment and to practise new skills; and
   (d) seeking out and being receptive to feedback.

3. I will help others make the most of their learning by:
   (a) providing feedback in constructive ways; and
   (b) contributing to the discussions about the experiences highlighted in the exercises.

4. I will use the theoretical input to learn from. This means I am willing to give serious consideration to the questions that are raised, to do additional reading, to participate in group discussions and to share my understanding with others in the group that our understanding of the nature of interpersonal relationships might be enriched. I will make the most of the experience of preparing and submitting work for assessment as a constructive learning exercise.

5. I will use professional judgement in keeping what happens among group members in the course appropriately confidential.

       Signed:

Note: No learning contract should be issued without discussion, and changes may be negotiated regarding content, wording, etc.

Exercise 1.1 Goals and expectations

Instructions

What do you hope to get from this course? What aspects of interpersonal skills do you want to concentrate your efforts on? What skills do you feel best about? What are the aspects of interpersonal skill which worry you or that you find difficult?

Please take time to think about these and any related questons that occur to you. Be as specific as possible, and in the interest of clarifying where you stand, make a brief written statement of your aims and objectives in taking the course. Make a summary of these below. This summary is for your own reference and you will not be asked to discuss it.

Answer sheet

My overall goal in this course is:

Some specific aspects of interpersonal skills I want to concentrate on are:

1.
2.
3.
4.
5.

I will have achieved my goals if, at the end of the course. I am able to:

1.
2.
3.
4.
5.

As you go through the course, your aims are likely to change. It is a good idea to repeat this exercise periodically and reassess your aims and achievements. Do keep all 'back copies' as they will provide you with a chart of your personal progress through the course.

Another means of recording progress and change is by keeping a diary/journal/log-book of interpersonal events. These can vary in the amount of detail recorded, and could take any form, such as those illustrated in Figure 1.3.

It has been suggested that records such as these can be included in the assessment/evaluation of student progress (see e.g. Ellis and Whittington's [1984] use of a log-book for evaluating health visitor training in interpersonal skills).

Whether or not any of these ideas are included as part of interpersonal skills learning, students should be encouraged to keep all course material (exercises and so on), and to look at it again regularly. This will give them some idea of their own progress and development.

1.3 Evaluation and assessment

Recording progress, as outlined above, may or may not contribute to assessment or evaluation. On thinking about measurements and evaluation a distinction must be made between the teaching and the learning.

Evaluation of teaching must be linked to the educational objectives that are established. If these are vague, evaluation too will be vague. If they are specific, evaluation must reflect this. On evaluating the teaching, both the content and the methods should be examined, and evaluators (usually teachers and/or students) should have a clear idea of how they will respond to their findings. In other words, will they modify content and/or methods in the light of the evaluation? Finding answers to the questions 'has it worked?', 'was it successful?', 'did it warrant the amount of time spent on it?', and so on is not easy, and is inevitably linked to issues of assessing and evaluating the learning. If nothing is learnt, the teaching has, presumably, been unsuccessful.

This raises, though, the problem of establishing learning criteria that must be met in order to assert that learning and teaching has succeeded. If, as we have argued, interpersonal skill is a continuing process and not an outcome, this becomes very difficult. We may well find that we are considering the distinction between *good* interpersonal skills and *good enough* interpersonal skills, acquired over a certain length of time (that is the length of interpersonal skills training). If, too, as we have argued, interpersonal skills are constrained by the context in which they are used, we are faced with the question of how

Figure 1.3 Samples of diary/journal/log formats

General

Setting: Female Medical

Date: 14.8.85

Interpersonal event: 4.30 p.m. I interrupted a visit to Mrs B. to ask about fluid balance.

Outcome: Mrs B. embarrassed. Annoyed with myself for insensitivity.

More detailed

Setting: Female Medical

Date: 14.8.85

Situation and People: 4.30 p.m. Mrs B. in bed. 2 visitors (1 male, 1 female). I interrupted and asked how much she had had to drink.

Outcome: Mrs B. embarrassed. Gave info. though. Visitors seemed startled.

My feelings: Annoyed at my insensitivity. Perplexed — need fluid balance information. How to get it with open visiting? Could have perhaps asked differently.

Critical incident

Setting: Female Medical

Date: 14.8.85

Incident: Info. re fluid balance from Mrs B.

Analysis:
Me: No introduction; multiple questions; no explanation; no reassurance; Mrs. B stopped talking to visitors

Mrs B: Asked for clarification. Gave information. Embarrassed.

Recommendation: Tell patients in advance that information will be required. Allow patient to record own intake in future? Explain why it's necessary and explain what constitutes fluid. All seems to revolve around patients understanding the need and being told in advance. This would avoid embarrassment in front of visitors.

to take account of this context when assessing individual levels of skill. A final consideration that must be made relates, again, to how the assessment information will be used. Many questions could be asked as such as: will students who are *not* good enough in terms of their interpersonal skills fail their training? Will those who are good enough in terms of their interpersonal skills with respect to one client group (say elderly people) be confined to the clientele in their professional practice? What attempts have been made in the interpersonal skills training to generalize the skills learnt to the assessment setting?

These are only some of the issues surrounding the interpretation of assessment information. (For further discussion of assessment and evaluation issues see Faulkner [1985]). Given the approach we have adopted to the nature of interpersonal skill, we would suggest that students should play a large part in evaluating their own learning, not with a view to 'failing' or 'succeeding', but in order to identify progress and gaps to fill in the future.

1.4 Summary

This chapter has been concerned with some of the issues facing tutors and students who are about to embark on an interpersonal skills course. Specifically the following issues were raised:

Interpersonal skills courses should meet the varying needs of different student groups.

Several questions need to be asked prior to mounting an interpersonal skills course.

Tutors vary in terms of interest and motivation, expertise and defensiveness.

Tutors should be encouraged to participate in some experiential learning.

Resources such as time, location, equipment, and personal support for tutors and students will influence the quality of interpersonal skills learning.

The context of an interpersonal skills course will depend on tutor/student experiences, resources and professional requirements.

Interpersonal skills teaching requires the use of experiential methods.

Experiential learning will only be of use if adequate preparation is made, and time given to processing student experiences and giving feedback.

Interpersonal skills courses and individual sessions should be structured carefully to link with students' other learning and life experiences.

The validity of interpersonal skills courses will depend on student needs, appropriate content and methods and the extent to which courses encourage the transfer of skills from one setting to another.

Students vary in terms of their own interpersonal skills, attitudes, motivation and level of self-confidence and consciousness.

Classes may be coherent or disparate in terms of the amount of similarity between students.

The experiential learning approach adopted here requires tutors to take a facilitative role.

Tutors have responsibility for creating a safe learning environment for students.

Students have responsibility to participate fully and honestly in sessions.

Learning contracts can be negotiated in order that students and tutors clarify their responsibilities at the outset.

Students should be encouraged to monitor their own progress and change.

Diaries are a useful method of monitoring progress and change.

Evaluation of interpersonal skills teaching should be linked to educational objectives.

Methods and content of teaching should be modified in the light of evaluation.

Learning criteria should be established if assessment is to be of value.

The role of assessment of interpersonal skills in the context of the rest of nurse training must be given serious consideration.

The nature of assessment and evaluation will depend to a certain extent on whether interpersonal skills acquisition is seen as a process or an outcome.

Students should be encouraged to participate in their own assessment.

Further reading

Ellis, R.A.F. and Whittington, D. (1981) *A Guide to Social Skill Training*, Croom Helm, London

Faulkner, A. (1985) The evaluation of teaching interpersonal skills to nurses. In C. Kagan (Ed.) *Interpersonal Skills in Nursing: Research and Applications*, Croom Helm, London

Kagan, C. (Ed.) (1985) Teaching interpersonal skills to nurses, *Interpersonal Skills in Nursing; Research and Applications*, Croom Helm, London, Part 5

McNulty, M. (1984) A framework for the future, *Nursing Mirror*, vol 158 (mental health forum supplement), pp i–iv

Tomlinson, A. (1985) The use of experiential methods in teaching interpersonal skills to nurses. In C. Kagan (Ed.) *Interpersonal Skills in Nursing; Research and Applications*, Croom Helm, London

CHAPTER 2

SELF-AWARENESS

As we saw in Figure I, self-awareness is central to interpersonal skill. We use knowledge about ourselves to plan our part in any interaction, and to put these plans into practice: our past experience contributes to our attitudes and values and affects *what* we notice about other people's behaviour, and how we interpret it. Understanding our reactions to what others say and do will help us relate more effectively to them. This is particularly so in a helping relationship. If, for example, a mastectomy patient wants to talk about her prognosis, we will be of little help if we have unacknowledged fear of mastectomy ourselves, or become distracted by the memory that someone close to us died of breast cancer. It is essential in any helping profession, including nursing, to have the opportunity to examine our reactions to what is happening in our daily work, throughout the course of our professional lives: self-awareness is not a 'once and for all' activity — it is a process that should be constantly reviewed.

Self-awareness can relate to any or all of the following:

(a) Personal identity, i.e. Who am I? How did I get to be who I am?
(b) Internal events, i.e. physiological sensations, thoughts, values, attitudes, beliefs, emotions.
(c) External events, i.e. behaviour, speech, membership of clubs, etc.
(d) Our sense of self as 'agent', i.e. the extent to which we believe we have control over the things that happen to us.

2.1 Personal identity

There is a view that 'self' is the essence of the adult personality, and that identity is formed as a result of significant events that have occurred during our childhood and adolescence. An alternative, but not incompatible view, is that we get a sense of our identity from the ways in which other people react towards us: this process continues throughout life. Thus the first approach suggests that our sense of identity in adulthood is quite stable, but the second approach suggests that identity is constantly susceptible to change. Exercise 2.1 is an exploration of personal identity.

Identity is inextricably linked to role, and the combination of roles that we occupy. The more pervasive the role(s), the greater is its contribution to identity. Thus, being a student nurse, living in the nurses' home, being friends with and going on holiday with other student nurses, will ensure that 'nurse' becomes an important feature of identity. Indeed, the very wearing of uniforms helps reduce visible signs of individuality, thus encouraging people to relate to us in terms of our *role* rather than as individual people (take, for example, the calling of 'nurse!', whichever nurse is on duty). Similarly, decking patients out in hospital issue nightgowns or pyjamas, all day and every day, removes *their* individuality, and helps increase the likelihood that they will identify with the role of patient. Often, when we think about ourselves, we think of those aspects we do not like, so some time to reflect on the *positive* parts of our identity is given in Exercise 2.2

2.2 Internal events

We learn to recognize and label internal bodily states through the guesses that adults make throughout our childhood. There is, therefore, enormous variation in our capacity to do so accurately. Sometimes, for all of us, our ability to recognize sensations breaks down. Consider, for example, feelings of nausea following sickness and diarrhoea: is it still the sickness or is it hunger that we are feeling? The context in which we experience the sensations partly determines the label we give to them. The case is similar for the labelling of emotional states. In general, the physiological changes underlying different emotional states are thought to be virtually indistinguishable. How then do we know whether we are excited, afraid, nervous, angry and so on? Take, for example, patients about to undergo surgery. They take their cues, firstly, from the thoughts they have ('I'll never recover from the anaesthetic');

Exercise 2.1   Explorations of personal identity

Instructions

Please work through the four sections of the exercise, answering all the questions as you go.

Answer sheet

1. In general, how introvert or extrovert would you say you were? (tick box)
Extremely   introvert: : : : : : : : : : : : : :   Extremely   extrovert

Imagine the centre of the circle is extremely introverted, and the edge of the circle is extremely extroverted, please mark how introverted/extroverted you would be in the different situations.

Mark on the chart how introverted/extroverted most other people would be in a comparable situation

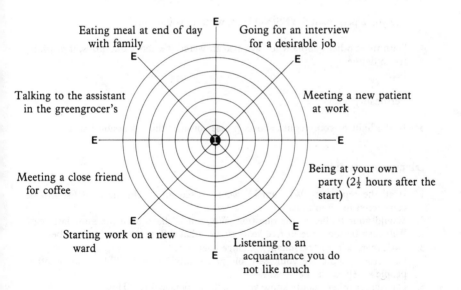

2. Please give twenty answers to the question 'Who am I?'

1.	11.
2.	12.
3.	13.
4.	14.
5.	15.
6.	16.
7.	17.
8.	18.
9.	19.
10.	20.

Now cross off any of these that are *descriptions* (e.g. I am fat, 19, popular, a Muslim, female, etc.). Cross off any that are *roles* (e.g. I am a student nurse, a daughter, a husband, a woman, etc.). You should be left with those replies that are unique to you as a person (such as I am Tom's wife, Mavis Roberts, me, my mother's son, etc.)

3. Please answer the following questions:
    Do you have a personality? YES/NO If so, please describe:

    Do you have personality? YES/NO If so, what do you mean?

    Are you a personality? YES/NO If so, what do you mean?

4. With three other people who have also answered the above questions, if possible, try to define
    Self:

    Personality:

5. In the light of your replies above, please consider the discussion issues.

Discussion issues

1. If all the replies to 'Who am I?' were crossed off, could the total list still be considered to be unique?
2. Would your replies to the question 'Who am I?' have been the same last year? Will they be the same in five years time? What differences might there be?
3. Do either 'self' or 'personality' change over time?
4. Can other people see your 'self' or 'personality'? Is it possible to know other people's 'selves' or 'personalities'?
5. Do you let other people know your 'self' or 'personality'? How?
6. How consistent is behaviour across different situations? What is it about situations that makes us behave differently in them?

Comments

---

secondly, from their behaviour ('Here I am reading every article I can find about the operation I am about to have'); and thirdly, from the social context ('staff in white coats are reassuring'). At times we may feel sensations that we are unable to identify, or we may even be unaware of the sensations themselves. Many training programmes that are designed to help people to reduce their level of anxiety contain elements to help them notice when they are becoming anxious or stressed so that they can take remedial action: in other words, they are being taught to be aware of internal events, and to label them appropriately.

Attitudes

Attitudes are internal events that are, too, difficult to label at times. Attitudes consist of positive or negative feelings and thoughts about an object, person or activity. So, statements such as 'I like Sister Brown,' 'I think disposable bedpans are a good thing,' 'I hate being on nights and think there should always be a qualified member of staff on every ward,' are all expressions of attitudes. Attitudes are, however, hypothetical constructs, in that they cannot be seen, and we simply infer them from what we feel, think and do. The relationship between attitudes and behaviour is an interesting one. What does it mean, for instance, if the nurse who says she likes Sister Brown runs and hides whenever she approaches; or the nurse who hails the advent of disposable bedpans always uses metal ones; or the student nurse who professes to dislike 'nights' and their organization always volunteers for extra night duty? What social meaning do attitudes have if we cannot predict behaviour from them?

Just as we can have attitudes towards other people (and we shall be considering *strong* attitudes towards others, or prejudices, and attempts to discourage them, in Chapter 7), so we can have attitudes towards ourselves. If

Exercise 2.2   Life histories: positive selves

Instructions

Take a large sheet of paper and draw the 'story of your life'. Spend about 20 minutes on this, bearing in mind the following rules:

Rules

1. The picture can take any form. Use as many colours as you wish.
2. Past events should be emphasized, but present circumstances and future hopes may be included.
3. The picture should culminate in a view of 'me as I am just now' with an emphasis on 'my strengths'.
4. Do not include anything you do not wish to.
5. There is no right or wrong way to do this.

With a group of colleagues who have also drawn the 'stories of their lives', if possible, discuss your pictures and consider the discussion issues.

Discussion issues

1. How many positive qualities did parents instill?
2. Has becoming a nurse developed any positive qualities?
3. How many positive qualities have come from personal choice?
4. Would your picture have been the same if it had been drawn for your parents or a group of good friends? Why/why not?
5. Was it easy to identify strengths? Why/why not?

Comments:

Exercise 2.3   Personal values and self-esteem

Instructions

1. Think of a person, living or dead, that you *most admire*, and write her/his name in the space provided.
2. Choose 6–10 characteristics that you admire this person for and list them down the left-hand side of the page.
3. On the rating scales, mark with a cross how much of each characteristic you think that person has/had.
4. Think of a person, living or dead, that you *least admire*, and write her/his name in the space provided.
5. On the rating scales, mark with a tick how much of each of the characteristics you think that person has/had.
6. Now think of *yourself*.
7. On the rating scales, mark with a circle how much of each of the characteristics you think you possess.

E.g. If you think the person you admire is very honest, but the person you least admire is not, and that you are also honest but not as honest as you could be, your ratings might look like this:

HONESTY	*High*				*Low*
: X :	. O :	:	./	:	:

Answer Sheet

Person most admired:
Person least admired:

Characteristics	*Ratings*
	High *Low*
1.	:___:___:___:___:___:___:___:
2.	:___:___:___:___:___:___:___:
3.	:___:___:___:___:___:___:___:
4.	:___:___:___:___:___:___:___:
5.	:___:___:___:___:___:___:___:
6.	:___:___:___:___:___:___:___:
7.	:___:___:___:___:___:___:___:
8.	:___:___:___:___:___:___:___:
9.	:___:___:___:___:___:___:___:
10.	:___:___:___:___:___:___:___:

The closer together the Xs and Os are, the higher the self-esteem

With a partner, discuss the extent to which you each have characteristics you value, and consider the discussion issues.

Discussion issues

1. Where did the characteristics you listed as admired or valued come from?
2. Do you think your best friend would have rated you differently? Why/why not?
3. How important are other people in making us feel good or bad about ourselves (that is, in giving us high or low self-esteem)?
4. Can self-esteem be raised or lowered? How?
5. How do you feel after doing this exercise?

Comments

---

we have a strong positive attitude towards ourselves (think highly of, and like ourselves), we are said to have *high self-esteem:* if we have a strong negative attitude towards ourselves (think badly of, and dislike ourselves) we are said to have *low self-esteem.* Most people are happier, and more confident in their daily lives if they have high self-esteem, and we shall see later that level of self-esteem can also be affected by our sense of self as 'agent'. The ways in which our personal values affect our self-esteem are highlighted in Exercise 2.3

One of the major ways in which we form attitudes towards ourselves, is to compare ourselves with others (see Exercise 2.3). How similar are we to those we like or to those we dislike? Sometimes we get an idea of someone, or a group of people we would like to be like, and then try to acquire the characteristics or behaviours that would make us more like them. So the child who wants to be a nurse will use 'nurses' as a reference group to provide information on how to act, and so on. Similarly, the nurse who had really wanted to be a doctor may try to act like one. (It is interesting to consider why some nurses, psychologists etc., who have a PhD call themselves 'Doctor' when they work in hospital settings: there is no reason why they should not — but what does doing so reveal about their concept of 'self'?)

Values and beliefs

In nursing, the values and beliefs we hold will affect the way we react to different situations. Values are generally thought to be central to our personal being, and to unify our behaviour. With reference to interpersonal skills, those values that arise from our desire to satisfy 'social needs' are particularly relevant. Our 'need to be liked' can lead to a sense of rejection if our efforts for particular patients do not appear to be appreciated: our 'need to be needed' may detract from our ability to discern patients' own needs if it makes us blinkered: our 'need for power' may mean that we act insensitively towards colleagues, and so on. Values, then, bring consistency to our behaviour, and are resistant to change. Any changes in values that do occur, however, will result in widespread changes of behaviour. Consider the way a colleague may change when there are prospects for promotion which highlight her/his need for power: she/he may well put on a different 'face' when senior personnel are present, adopt positions she/he had not previously held and even cut off long standing friendships.

Some beliefs, too, are thought to be central and highly resistant to change. When these beliefs do change, the effects for the person are often traumatic, and they influence all aspects of behaviour. Others may be far more inconsequential, easily changed and have no widespread effects. The different types of beliefs, with examples, are shown on Table 2.1, and Exercise 2.4 focuses on the nature of beliefs about nursing.

2.3 External events

On the whole, we are aware of how we talk and behave, which clubs we belong to and why. What we may not be aware of is the information these external events give other people about our own identity. It is often said that we each have 'public' and 'private' selves: we take care to present our 'public' selves in ways that give different information to different groups of people. The book we choose to read on the train, the clothes we choose to wear to party or a job interview, the way we greet the nursing officer, will all reveal different aspects of our 'self' to the different audiences. The more involved in a role we are (with all the attendant 'props', like uniforms — again!), the less personal information we reveal. Thus it is hard to get to know much about the way individual patients really think and feel if they are fully immersed in the patient role. (An optimistic view of the nursing process is that if it is

Table 2.1 Types of belief and consequences of change

Type of belief	Source of belief	Example	Change
Shared primitive beliefs	Widely held in a particular culture	I believe in the sanctity of life	Difficult — leading to trauma
Unshared primitive beliefs	Self-identity and personal experience	I believe men should have equal responsibility for child care	Difficult — leading to widespread changes
Authority beliefs	Derived from (perceived) legitimate authority (e.g. the hospital authorities)	I believe staffing levels in the N.H.S. should be maintained (after all it's district policy)	Can change with perceived legitimacy of the authority or with changing experiences
Derived beliefs	Derived from authorities with which individual identifies (e.g. another valued person)	I believe in giving patients the option to have electroconvulsive shock treatment. (That's what my tutor believes)	Can change with changing experiences, and often through communication
Inconsequential beliefs	Past experience, prejudices, etc.	I believe this ward always gets the post last	Easily changed. No pervasive effects.

Source: After M. Rokeach, *Beliefs, Attitudes and Values*, Jossey-Bass, Beverley Hills, CA, 1968

Exercise 2.4   Beliefs about nursing

Instructions

With reference to Table 2.1, please think of your own beliefs. List as many beliefs you hold about nursing as you can. Try to identify the source of these beliefs, and thus the type of belief each represents, i.e.

shared primitive belief, unshared primitive belief, authority belief, derived belief, and inconsequential belief.

Answer sheet

Belief	Source	Type
I believe ...	I acquired this belief from ...	

In the light of your replies, please consider the discussion issues.

Discussion issues

1. Were any of the beliefs easier to identify than others? Why might this be?
2. How susceptible to change do you think your beliefs are?
3. Are some people's belief systems more rigid than others? Are these people more predictable than others?
4. Is there anything about nurse education that attempts to change beliefs about nursing? Please identify.

Comments

implemented effectively, role barriers should be broken down to allow access to people as *people*, not as 'patients', 'nurses' etc.).

Self-presentation

Sociologists have written extensively on the attempts we make to present our 'self' in a particular light. It is as if we are all actors on a stage, playing roles at all times, however informally, to different audiences, depending on the situation. Extending the analogy with the theatre, we all have 'front' and 'backstage' areas: we perform publicly in order to give particular impressions to our 'audience' when we are frontstage, but drop the 'mask' when we return to the more private backstage. In this vein, the nurses who behave with bristling efficiency on the ward to the 'audience' of patients, and who collapse in exhausted heaps when they believe themselves to be alone in the office, only to become dynamic when going on the ward again, are treating the ward as frontstage, and the office as backstage. As soon as anyone else walks into the office, they will quickly try to regain a frontstage appearance. The argument, then, is that we try to present facets of 'self' in different lights on different occasions. Our choice of how we do this depends largely on how we perceive ourselves, that is, the kind of person we think we are, and would like other people to think we are. It does not always happen like this: sometimes we try to hide the kind of person we think we are by presenting ourselves in particular ways. Even if we present ourselves in ways that are 'not really us', other people's reactions may mean that we start to become like that after all.

It can sometimes be surprising to find out what kind of a person other people think we are. Generally, we pick up cues about the impression we make on others from the way they behave towards us, but it can certainly be illuminating to be told. People's perceptions of us, and our impressions of others are explored in Exercises 2.5 and 2.6.

Subjective and objective self-awareness

To say that we think carefully about the ways we present ourselves to others is not to imply that we are continually self-aware. Certainly, when we are deciding what to wear one day, or are thinking about how happy or upset we might be, we are in state of self-awareness. We are *subjectively self-aware*, in so far as we are aware of internal events. Every now and then, though, something

Exercise 2.5 Self-perception and feedback from others

Instructions

This exercise is a group exercise. It cannot be done individually. If you cannot find a group of people with whom to participate, read through the instructions carefully, and try to imagine what might have happened if you had been able to 'play the game'. In groups of 6–12 (no larger if possible), play the following game:

Procedure

1. Sit round in a circle, as comfortably as possible. Each person is to think about another person in the group, and to think of that characteristic that most aptly describes him/her (this can be an internal or an external characteristic, that is to do with attitudes, values, beliefs, temperament or appearance etc.).
2. When everyone has thought of one, the first person announces the characteristic she/he was thinking of, *without* saying who it referred to. Everyone else is to think whether she/he is being referred to. If anyone thinks the characteristic applies to her/him, ask *'Is it me?'* She/he is then told whether it was she/he that was in mind.
3. If it was not she/he that was in mind, the first person says 'No'. Anyone else that thinks the characteristic refers to her/him then asks if it is she/he that is in mind. If three people claim the characteristic incorrectly, the first person tells the group who she/he was thinking of.
4. As soon as someone rightly claims the characteristic, or the first person tells the group who she/he had been thinking of, the next person sitting in an anti-clockwise position announces the characteristic she/he has in mind, and the process is continued.
5. The procedure is repeated until everyone in the circle has announced the characteristic she/he had in mind. It does not matter if different people in the group had thought of a characteristic and/or person that somebody else had already announced. If possible, members should stick with the characteristic/person they had first thought of.
6. The game can be repeated until members can no longer think of characteristics, or until time permits.

When the game is over, it is vital that some time is spent discussing participants' experiences. Together, consider the Discussion issues. If there has been any conflict in the discussion, try to deal with it before terminating the session.

Discussion issues

1. How easy was it to know whether the characteristics referred to oneself?

2. Were members inhibited about claiming characteristics? If so, why?
3. Did anyone feel that another person's perception of her/him was surprising? Why?
4. Was there anyone who was not named at all? If so, how does she/he feel about this?
5. Was there anyone who was 'chosen' a lot? If so, how does she/he feel about this?
6. How do discrepancies between how we think about ourselves and how other people see us arise?
7. What kinds of decisions did members make in choosing the characteristics of others? (For example, did they choose obvious ones, 'safe' ones, complimentary ones, hurtful ones, etc.?) Would the decisions about which characteristics to choose have been different if this were not a party game rather than a class activity? Why/Why not?
8. Is there anything else anyone would like to say about the exercise?

Comments

Exercise 2.6 Perceptions of known and unknown others

Instructions

Select some pictures of unknown and well-known people In groups of four (if possible) examine each picture in turn and discuss answers to the following questions. Try to come to some agreement.

1. What do you think this person does and why?
2. What do you think this person is like as a person and why?
3. Do you think you would like this person? Why/why not?

Answer sheet

Person 1 (known/unknown*)
1.
2.
3.
Person 2 (known/unknown*)
1.
2.
3.
Person 3 (known/unknown*)
1.
2.
3.
Person 4 (known/unknown*)
1.
2.
3.
* Delete as appropriate

When you have completed your explorations of the four people, consider the discussion issues.

Discussion issues

1. How did prior experience or knowledge affect the answers to the questions? Was there agreement amongst group members with respect to the well-known people?
2. On what basis do we generally form impressions of others? What cues did you use to make your decisions about the stimulus pictures?
3. How easily changed are these judgements?
4. Is it possible to identify characteristics that are always liked or disliked in others?
5. How do values affect our perceptions of and judgements about other people?
6. What differences were there in the cues used to make judgements about known and unknown people?

Comments

happens to make us aware of ourselves as other people see us: we are then *objectively self-aware*. When we catch sight of ourselves in a shop window, see a photograph or hear a tape-recording of ourselves, we are thrown into a state of objective self-awareness ('Is that how I appear to other people?'). When we are, or think we are, being watched or examined, we are also thrown into a state of objective self-awareness ('What would Sister think of the way I am giving this injection?'). One of the consequences of being made objectively self-aware is that we become aware of our deficiencies, and are likely to make a decision to change in some way ('I must get a hair-cut, go on a diet, watch my accent, talk to the patient, etc.) People differ, though, in how far they are aware of either internal or external events: some people are painfully aware of themselves and their shortcomings and are likely to be self-conscious as a result: others are impervious to even their largest 'imperfections', and certainly to others' reactions to them, and they may well be arrogant and over self-confident. Happily, most of us compromise between realistic self-appraisal and the motivation to change some aspects of our 'selves'. As nurses, positive feedback from people that coincides with how *we* feel about ourselves will make us feel good and enjoy our work: negative feedback from others that contradicts how we see ourselves will make us miserable and dissatisfied with work. Ironically, the public's expectations of nurses frequently contradicts our own perception of the nursing role: this becomes more apparent to students as they progress through training, and often contributes to increasing dissatisfaction with the job. Similarly, the mismatch between patient's expectations of nurses in, say, intensive care settings (to make comfortable and to reassure, etc.) with the nurses' tasks of administering some painful treatment (such as coughing and aspiration after thoracic surgery) may lead to dissatisfaction.

2.4 Sense of self as 'agent'

We have seen, above, that our feelings about ourselves are determined, in part, by the ways in which other people react towards us. Furthermore, we try to control the impression they get of us by presenting ourselves in particular ways. In order to have self-confidence and to act effectively, we must hold the belief that we *can* control how others see us. In addition, we must hold a belief that we are able to have some control over our environment. In other words, we have to believe in ourselves as 'agents', and not as objects to be controlled by others. If we experience little or no control over our environment, our health and morale may decline, leading to illness, depression and even, it is suggested, death. However, it is the *belief* that we have control, rather than the control itself, that leads to psychological and physical well-being, self-confidence and high self-esteem, which in turn increases our ability to be effective in our personal relationships.

Perceived lack of control

Perceived lack of control, leading to the passivity described above, is characteristic of people who are ill, and who think there is nothing they can do about it. A different effect is found if people think they *should* be able to control their health: they may react against their apparent lack of control and 'fight', displaying what is known as 'reactance'. Reactance can occur whenever we find ourselves unable to control events that we expect to be able to, or when we think that we are being denied freedom of choice. So we can evoke the concept of reactance to understand the obese patient's eating binges when she/he has been put on a diet: her/his freedom of choice is restricted, albeit for her/his own good. The binge is an attempt to regain control.

Perceived lack of control leads to stress, and the different reactions we all have to lack of control is partly due to our different reactions to stress. Working in a context where we are unable to decide anything for ourselves is likely to be stressful, and we will experience a weak sense of self as 'agent'. Hospitals are wonderful places for denying patients and staff alike the choice over all manner of things to do with their daily life. Consider a long stay ward: patients cannot choose how to place their furniture, (sometimes) what they can have on top of their locker, whether to get up or stay in bed, (sometimes) what to have to eat (even if they ostensibly have a choice of menu, their 'order' does not always arrive), when to have a bath, what to wear and so on. Staff may not be able to choose when to talk to a particular patient (or when not to), when to have a cup of tea, what to wear, what to do, and so on; consequently they may leave at the end of the day feeling as though they have been shoved around all day and that they are a 'nobody'. Not only is it important, then, that we retain some sense of self as 'agent' in order to remain psychologically healthy ourselves, but we should remember to give *others* the opportunity to experience themselves as 'agents', too.

The processes involved in the different reactions to perceived lack of control are shown in Figure 2.1, and are illustrated in Exercise 2.7.

Figure 2.1 Consequences of real/perceived lack of control for self-esteem: sense of self as 'agent'

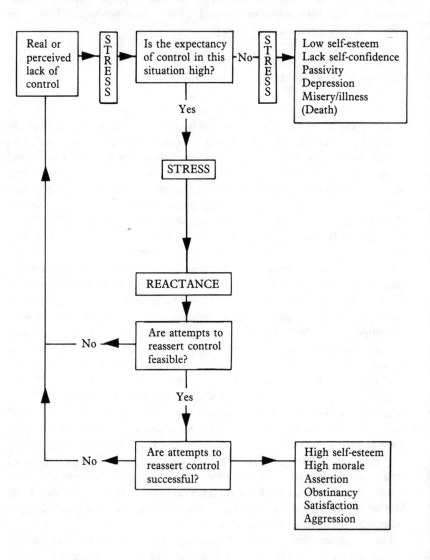

Exercise 2.7   Self as 'agent' and lack of control

Instructions

Please read Chapter 2 and make sure you are familiar with the material. Think of a recent event which resulted in you (a) becoming passive, and (b) displaying reactance.

Answer sheet

For each situation describe:

1. The circumstances that led up to it:
   (a)

   (b)

2. The attempts (if any) you made to regain control:
   (a)

   (b)

3. What the consequences were for your self-esteem:
   (a)

   (b)

4. Why attempts to regain control either did or did not work:
   (a)

   (b)

5. Whether this reaction was typical or not, and if not, why you responded in this way:
   (a)

   (b)

When you have completed these analyses, consider the discussion issues either by yourself or with others who have also completed the exercise.

Discussion issues

1. Would your reaction have been the same if the other main people involved had been of the opposite sex/20 years older/from a different culture, etc.? Why/why not?
2. How important was the specific situation in making you react in the way you did? In what ways?

Comments:

The importance of self as 'agent' is a product of a culture where an individual's freedom of choice and expression is highly valued. It is interesting to consider how prominently self as 'agent' features in other cultures and/or subcultures. Do people from different cultures react differently to being asked to cooperate in treatments, ward routines, not eating pre-operatively, and so on? Is reactance common to all cultures and subcultures? It follows from the above discussion that people who are used to having a lot of power/control will react most strongly to loss of control. If this is so, we might expect teachers, company directors, politicians and doctors, for example, to make particularly 'bad' patients; furthermore, they should be at their worst when they are feeling relatively well, but some restrictions are imposed upon them (for example on enforced immobility following orthopaedic surgery). Does experience bear this out?

2.5 The process of becoming self-aware

We said earlier that self-awareness was not achieved once and for all, but rather that it was a continuing process. It can be argued that one of the main purposes of life is to strive for a state of 'self-actualisation', and self-awareness is one of the means we have for achieving this. We become healthier and happier if we can be aware of ourselves and be open and honest in our transactions with other people. Only when we are able to do this, and to integrate all our experiences – past, present and future – into our self-system, will we be able to help others effectively. It is not supposed that increased self-awareness will lead us all to become paragons of virtue. Instead, we should be able to use the knowledge we have about our shortcomings, fears, preferences, and so on, so that we can see when our concerns with 'self' are obstructing our ability to help our clients/patients/friends etc. We can only remove the obstructions when we are able to recognize them in the first place. Self-awareness comes about largely through our relations with other people, and the process is usefully summed up in Figure 2.2

We will never achieve total self-awareness (how would we know we had achieved it?), but can work at making constructive use of our experiences throughout life, in order to enhance our personal relationships and make more effective use of our interpersonal skills.

2.6 Summary

This chapter has outlined some of the ways in which self-awareness underlies effective use of interpersonal skills. Specifically, the following issues were raised:

Self-awareness is central to interpersonal skills.

Increased self-awareness leads to more effective use of interpersonal skills.

Self-awareness is a process that should constantly be under review.

Identity is acquired from various sources, and may become stable in adulthood.

Identity is inextricably linked to role.

Awareness of essential states depends on the context in which they are experienced.

Attitudes are hypothetical constructs and may or may not be closely linked to behaviour.

Attitudes towards 'self' determine levels of self-esteem.

Comparisons with other people help form attitudes towards 'self'.

Figure 2.2 The process of self-awareness through self-knowledge and feedback from other people: the Johari Window

	Known to Self	*Unknown to self*
Known to others	**a** *Public Self* What I know and I present to others so that they know it too.	**b** *Blind Self* Those aspects of me that I am unaware of but that others see and judge me by
Unknown to others	**c** *Private self* What I know but I do not want other people to know or to discover	**d** *Unknown self* What I do not know, or do not (want to) recognize, and that others are not aware of

The process of self-awareness means that those aspects known to 'self' are increased. Sometimes, the 'Private' area will also be decreased, for example:

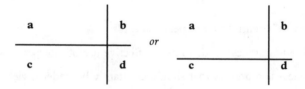

Values unify, and bring consistency to, social behaviour.

Values and beliefs are resistant to change.

Changes in beliefs may have traumatic consequences for the 'self'.

The presentation of 'public' and 'private' selves gives different information to different people.

Different facets of the 'self' are shown in different lights on different occasions.

Self-presentation is linked to self-perception.

Self-awareness may be objective or subjective.

Objective self-awareness often leads to change.

Belief in 'self as agent' leads to self-confidence and high self-esteem.

Perceived lack of control over events can lead to stress, passivity/depression or reactance.

Reactance leads to attempts to regain control and thereby to raise self-esteem.

Cultures vary in the importance they give to the belief in 'self as agent'.

Self-awareness comes largely from relations with other people.

Further reading

Gahagan, J. (1984) Knowledge and experience of self, *Social Interaction and its Management*, Methuen, London, Ch.7

Goffman, E. (1956) *The Presentation of Self in Everyday Life*, Anchor Books, New York (Pelican Edition, 1971)

Jourard, S. (1971) *Self Disclosure: An Experimental Analysis of the Transparent Self*, Wiley, New York

Rogers, C. (1961) *On Becoming a Person*, Houghton Mifflin, Boston, Mass.

Skevington, S. (1984) *Understanding Nurses*, Wiley, London

Smith, V.M. and Bass, T.A. (1982) Discovering yourself as the communicator, *Communication for the Health Care Team*, Harper and Row, London, Ch.2

CHAPTER 3

EXPLORATIONS IN INTERPERSONAL BEHAVIOUR

If we are to use effective interpersonal skills we must engage in social behaviour. It can be useful to consider both verbal and non-verbal aspects of social behaviour (see Figure I), although it is essential to remember that in most cases the two 'systems' are interrelated in complex ways. At times, though, one system may be dominant. In noisy environments, or when relating to people who have lost their hearing, permanently or temporarily, the non-verbal channel assumes dominance: in those situations where vision is attenuated, or permanently lost, the verbal channel assumes dominance. Sometimes, too, when ambiguous messages are given out (that is the person says something, but her/his body 'says' the opposite), one or other channel will be noticed more, depending on the situation. Just as the distinction between channels can be drawn in relation to behaviour, so it can be when we consider observation and the interpretation of other people's behaviour.

In order to make 'good' observations, it is necessary to be aware of the elements of both non-verbal and verbal behaviour that, combined, produce social behaviour.

3.1 Non-verbal behaviour

We use the term non-verbal behaviour here to refer to anything about social performance that is not speech, or the actual words that are spoken. We have said, above, that under normal circumstances non-verbal communication is not a separate communication system. Rather, it relates to speech in several different ways: non-verbal messages may enhance, replace (as in sign language), or contradict verbal messages. It is usually the non-verbal cues that we notice first, on meeting people, and on the basis of this information we form impressions about the other person's values and attitudes, personality, interests, and so on. In fact we make judgements very quickly about the kind of person we think she or he is. (We shall see later [Section 3.3] that these judgements may or may not be correct, but we make them nevertheless!) At the same time, we are giving a lot of information to others that may lead them to make judgements about our own values and attitudes etc. What are the cues that we respond to? (See Exercise 3.1).

It is likely that some, if not all, of the different categories of non-verbal behaviour, as shown in Table 3.1, will have been listed.

No attempt was made, in Exercise 3.1, to interpret the meaning of the different non-verbal behaviours. Generally, we assume that all behaviour means something, and react accordingly. We usually base our decisions about meaning on what we would *expect* the behaviour to mean, given the particular cultural and situational context in which it occurred. We may be wrong, of course, and the person we think is miserable just has 'that kind of face', or the person we think is nervous habitually looks past others when engaging them in conversation. Exercise 3.2 gives us some insight into the consequences of changing certain non-verbal habits.

Non-verbal habits

As we saw in Chapter 1, one assumption behind viewing interpersonal behaviour as a *skill* is that it is learnt. Thus we have learnt to behave in particular ways non-verbally (and verbally), usually responding differently in different situations. What we display at any particular point in time may be a *habit*, rather than a meaningful communication. The trouble is, of course, that we may not mean anything by a particular behaviour, but someone else might notice it and attach meaning to it. Similarly, we may judge other people's behaviour in certain ways that turn out to be totally inappropriate. The other thing to note about our 'habitual' ways of behaving is that they are difficult to change. They have built up over a long period of time, and it is not so easy to say, for example, 'Right, I must look at people more when they are speaking to me, in order to make them feel more at ease.' Once we try to change any part of our interpersonal skill, the system as a whole may be

Exercise 3.1   Taxonomy of non-verbal behaviour

Instructions

This exercise can be done individually, or with a partner.

Individual

Watch someone talking to someone else. Note down all the non-verbal behaviours they display. If you can, stand within earshot so that you can hear the tone of voice, pitch, etc. Write down as many non-verbal behaviours as you can in the chart below. If you need to, refer to Table 3.1 for reminders of the different non-verbal behaviours.

Collaborative

1. Allocate the roles A and B. Have a short conversation about the kinds of houses you live in (about 3 minutes). Note as many non-verbal behaviours that your partner displays, and write them in the chart below.
2. A — leave the room. B — stand in a space not too close to a wall. A — return to the room and have a conversation with B about good places to eat out (about 3 minutes). Again, note down the non-verbal behaviours displayed by your partner. Let your partner know what non-verbal behaviours you have noted.
3. Now sit back to back. Talk about those aspects of school or your last job that you liked the best. Note down any non-verbal behaviours. When you have carried out all three conversations, draw up a comprehensive list of non-verbal behaviours and discuss your experiences with reference to the discussion issues.

Answer sheet

Task:

List all the non-verbal cues you noticed, in the following categories:

Facial expression

Gesture (hand/head)

Proximity and touch (others and self)

Eye gaze

Posture, orientation and gait

Vocal

Artefacts

Discussion issues

1. Were the non-verbal behaviours you noticed linked in any way to the topic of conversation? If so, how? ·
2. Were you surprised at any of the non-verbal behaviours your partner noticed about you?
3. What nursing interactions are similar to the three different interactions in the collaborative exercise?
4. How is non-verbal behaviour used to best effect in nursing?
5. Would different non-verbal behaviours have been displayed by people who were older/younger? What differences would there have been?

Comments

Table 3.1   A taxonomy of non-verbal behaviour

Facial expression

Eyebrows	Nose	Cheeks
Forehead	Mouth	Eye movements
Eye region	Mouth region	Tongue

Gesture

Hand	Head shake, nod, toss	Facial
Arm	Body	Leg/foot
Vocal		

Proximity and touch
Patterns of bodily accessibility
Personal distance
Ritual/task-related physical contact
Touching self (scratching, rubbing, twiddling hair/rings, etc.)

Eye gaze

Eye contact	Staring	Avoidance
Direction of gaze	Duration of gaze	Blinking

Posture, orientation and gait
Position of limbs/head
Position of body
Regularity of movements
Speed/regularity walking

Vocal

Tone and pitch	Volume	Speed
Clarity	Amount	Silence
Pauses	Hesitations	Verbal cliches
Dysfluencies	Sighs	Laughs

Artefacts
Appearance: dress, cosmetics, hair, accessories (e.g. bags, spectacles, jewellery,),
   cleanliness, smell
Emblems: badges, uniforms, possessions (make of car, newspaper, etc.)

Note: Combinations of non-verbal behaviours mean different things, and *movement* changes the meaning.

Exercise 3.2   Habits and change

Instructions

This exercise should be carried out in groups of three.

1. In groups of three, allocate roles A, B and O (observer). A and B please think about your own non-verbal behaviour and decide to change any *two* aspects of it. Do not tell each other what you are going to change.
2. A and B have a brief conversation about the kinds of animals you like and dislike, whilst concentrating on changing those two aspects of your non-verbal behaviour, previously decided. O — take notes on anything you notice about the interaction between A and B. Throughout the conversation, O should remind A and B to concentrate on changing their non-verbal behaviours.
3. After about 4 minutes, stop the conversation, and tell each other which non-verbal behaviours your partner was changing. O — give feedback to both A and B regarding their interaction.

At the end of the feedback session, continue your discussion about the exercise with reference to the discussion issues.

Discussion issues

1. What happened to the conversation?
2. What was it like as speaker, listener and observer?
3. Were the changes in non-verbal behaviours correctly identified? If not, why not?
4. Did any unintended changes in the interaction occur? (such as other non-verbal changes, conversation drying up, not hearing the other person, etc.) If so, what does this say about the strength of learning non-verbal behaviours?
5. How easy is it to change habitual non-verbal behaviours?
6. How can you distinguish between meaningful non-verbal behaviours and habits?

Comments

affected, as we saw in Exercise 3.2. Still, it is worth trying to change those habits of ours that we know detract from effective use of interpersonal skills, but we should bear in mind (and be prepared to deal with) the other (unintended) changes that may occur.

Encounter regulation

Non-verbal behaviour is of critical importance in the regulation of encounters. By this, we mean encouraging others to speak, ensuring that they remain silent while we speak, and so on. In addition, it is the non-verbal behaviours that convey to others our feelings of dominance or subordination, or just generally make us feel at ease or uncomfortable. The extent to which this is so can be seen if we consider the quality of interactions on the telephone, as compared with face-to-face conversations. On the telephone, neither party can see the other; interruptions are frequent, and the normal course of the conversation is disrupted (how many of us have experienced the total impossibility of ending a telephone conversation?). All of this is largely because the non-verbal information we have is limited to vocal cues. In telephone conversations, most non-verbal cues are eliminated for both people: there are, however, many situations where one person has more information about non-verbal cues than the other. In such cases, rather different effects on the interaction are felt, as we can see from Exercise 3.3.

The person who has more non-verbal information will usually dominate the conversation. There are very many nursing situations wherein the nurse has greater access to non-verbal information than her/his patient — or rather the patient has less access to non-verbal information than the nurse. Lying down while someone talks to us from the end of the bed is one very common example. More obviously, perhaps, is the person who has a visual handicap, a hearing deficiency, or, due to some dressing or medical procedure is temporarily deprived of hearing/sight etc. These encounters make it very easy for the nurse to dominate the conversation, a theme we will return to later.

In subsequent sections, we will be considering the use of non-verbal behaviours in the communication of emotion and interpersonal attitudes (Sections 5.2, 5.3), the regulation of encounters and the emphasis of speech (Sections 3.2, 6.1) and in complex interpersonal settings, such as counselling (Chapter 5) and those requiring assertion (Chapter 6). We will now consider in some detail the role of language in interpersonal skill: the use of speech is, however, inextricably linked to certain aspects of non-verbal behaviour, particularly those in the 'paralinguistic' category.

Exercise 3.3   Encounter regulation

Instructions

1. With a partner, sit back to back at the normal distance for holding a conversation. Discuss the merits of different kinds of food for 3–5 minutes. Note down, without discussing it, what this felt like for each of you.
2. Sit opposite each other at normal conversational distance. One person put on a blindfold (a scarf or a handkerchief would do). Assume you are planning a holiday: please discuss where and when to go for 3–5 minutes. Note down, without discussing it, what this felt like for each of you.
3. Together, or with other people who have also carried out the exercise, share your experiences and consider the discussion issues.

Discussion issues

1. Who talked the most in each conversation? Why?
2. Are there any nursing situations where one person can see the other but not vice versa? Please give examples.
3. In such situations, can you think of any ways that the 'sighted' person can help her/his partner feel more comfortable and 'equal' in the conversation?

Comments

3.2 Speech

We can consider the elements of speech at a number of different levels, from sounds, syllables, words, phrases, sentences, to sequences, and so on. For our purposes here, we will examine the social use of language, and so consider it at the level of meaning. As with non-verbal behaviour, there may well be a mismatch between what the speaker intended and what the listener thought she/he meant. Most things we say have both *latent* (hidden) and *manifest* (obvious) meanings. For example:

> 'What was that you said?'
> *Manifest:* 'Please repeat what you said'.
> *Latent:* 'You're so boring, I wasn't listening'.

Cues as to which meaning is *intended* are given by the expression we use and other non-verbal accompaniments, such as facial expression and timing. So, at times we can *intend* the latent meaning to be picked up, and confusion will arise if the listener responds to the manifest meaning; at other times, however, we may intend the manifest meaning, but the listener interprets what we say at the latent level, once more leading to confusion. Smooth interaction requires both listener and speaker to be operating at the same level of meaning (see Figure 3.1).

As we shall see later, many of the strategies of speech we use exploit the ambiguity inherent in the two levels of meaning.

Rules of conversations

A great deal of what we say (and how we interpret what others say) is in accordance with *rules*. These rules, which may be explicit (clearly stated) or implicit (assumed), determine the level of detail that is used, the content of what is said, the order of successive bits of speech and how the elements are related to each other. There are some general rules that govern many different aspects of interaction, but there are also rules that are specific to different situations and the roles people occupy in those situations. Let us take an informal conversation as example. We will generally abide by the following rules:

Figure 3.1   Interaction as a function of shared level of meaning

Interaction	Smooth	Disrupted
Speaker intends Listener perceives	LATENT LATENT	LATENT MANIFEST
Speaker intends Listener perceives	MANIFEST MANIFEST	MANIFEST LATENT

(a) Each participant has the chance to talk.
(b) Only one person speaks at one time.
(c) Gaps between utterances are brief.
(d) The order of speaking is not fixed in advance.
(e) Utterances frequently follow 'rules of relevance', such as
    (i)   question — answer,
    (ii) statement — acknowledgement,
    (iii) offer — acceptance/refusal,
    (iv) apology — acknowledgement/rejection.

If any of these rules are broken, the interaction will be disrupted, and confusion may arise. However, the rules are not invariant, and both partners may not be fully aware of them. Furthermore, they are often (sub)culturally specific, and may change with the situation, as illustrated in Exercise 3.4.

The breaking of the rules of conversation is often an attempt to communicate something that we find difficult to say. This nurse, for example, is sensitive to the underlying message being given by the patient as she/he breaks the rules of conversation:

Nurse: What did you have for dinner?
Patient: They've changed my pills. (*Breaking rule of relevance.*)
Nurse: Oh? Does that worry you? (*Sensitive response.*)
Patient: I … yes … well … I think it does … I mean, I must be getting worse, aren't I?

Exercise 3.4   Rules of conversations

Instructions

1. Choose a conversation from the list below and write the rules underlying it on a sheet of paper.
2. Repeat this for all the conversations.
3. List the rules for the same conversations as if they were taking place with someone 20 years older than the other (make it clear who is the older person).
4. Show a friend or colleague the list of conversations and explain briefly to her/him the notion that all conversations have rules for conducting them, that both partners generally follow. Show her/him one of your lists of rules and ask her/him if she/he can link these rules to one of the conversations on the list.

Conversations

1. Patient assessment.
2. Counselling.
3. Explaining an operative procedure.
4. Giving bad news to a relative.
5. Consoling a patient whose mother is late visiting.
6. Explaining why a middle-aged woman should not sit on her bed with her ankles crossed.
7. Telling a colleague of suspected fetal distress during delivery within earshot of the mother.
8. As an infection control specialist, asking the ward sister for her cooperation.
9. Gaining access to a patient's house for the first time in the community.

Discuss the problems of correctly identifying the conversations from the rules, and consider the discussion issues.

Discussion issues

1. Were some of the conversations more difficult to identify from their rules than others? Why might this be?
2. What difference did the age make to the conversation rules? Why?
3. Did role or setting influence the rules of the conversation? If so, how?
4. Are there any nursing situations that do not have rules underlying the conversations? Please describe.
5. Are the rules of a conversation the same for everyone who is talking? What differences might there be for patients and nurses in some of the above examples?

Comments

This nurse, on the other hand, is insensitive:

Nurse: What did you have for dinner?
Patient: They've changed my pills. (*Breaking rule of relevance.*)
Nurse: You were meant to have had cod in cheese sauce. (*Persisting, insensitive.*)
Patient: What? ... Oh, yes. We did.

Sometimes, just listening to or reading *what* was said is misleading, as the rules of relevance may appear to have been broken, but are, in fact, unspoken, but fully understood by both participants. For example:

Patient: Can I walk to the bathroom?
Nurse: Sister will be here in a minute.

This seems to be an insensitive response by the nurse, but when we know, as both patient and nurse do here, that sister has said she wants to go with this patient when she/he walks to the bathroom, we see that the rules of relevance had not been broken, and that the nurse was responding appropriately. This illustrates rather well the need to be aware of the *context* in which conversations take place, in order fully to understand them.

Strategies of speech

Factors determining what we say and how we say it, then, depend to a large extent on the rules prescribed by the situation. The more formal the situation, the greater the constraints on who says what to whom. Weddings, committees, and so on are examples of formal situations with predetermined rules of speech. Such regular patterns of speech, that are clearly dictated by rules, are known as *rituals*, and will be considered in greater detail in Chapter 4. They apply, as we shall see, to less formal situations as well as the formal ones.

There are other social and interpersonal considerations that determine our choice of language, most of which are linked in some way to the roles we and our partner(s) fulfil.

The style of speech we adopt is known as the 'code', and reflects the assumptions we make about (what we take to be) the listener's state of knowledge. For example, the request 'Please take this to her, over there,' assumes that the listener knows what is to be taken to whom, and the context is such that the person's whereabouts is known. Another request, however, makes no such assumption: 'Please take this haemoglobin report to Sister — she is the one in blue who is standing over by the window.' The first request was made in a *restricted code* (RC) and the second in an *elaborated code* (EC). An 'outsider' would not be able to understand the RC as it assumes a great deal of prior knowledge. Talking 'shop' and using jargon are further examples of RC, and they are frequently used to convey the message, 'You are not one of us.' It can be embarrassing, and even humiliating, to have to ask for elaboration of a RC, as this is tantamount to saying, 'I am not familiar with you/the subject/the situation.' Consider, for example, the following:

Patient: Nurse, it's time I went now. (*Restricted code.*)
Nurse: Went where? (*Request for elaboration.*)
Patient (to other patient): Wouldn't you know it? Just my luck — a new 'un!
  (*Consequences for relationship.*)

Explanations, or conversations with strangers, often have to be made in EC. Exercise 3.5 explores the value of EC when communication is limited.

Relative power and status of partners is reflected by the form of address we use (see Chapter 4), and also by, for example, who is permitted to initiate conversations. So, on a ward round, a 'rule' may be that the consultant can address a student nurse, but not vice versa. The 'high status' person, then, has the right to control the interaction.

We have seen that the level of precision used, reflects what the speaker thinks the listener needs to know. Using RC like this can, however, lead the listener to make incorrect inferences from what is said. This can be illustrated by the following conversation:

Nurse 1: Jane stayed in bed all day yesterday. (*Making assumptions about listener's state of knowledge.*)
Nurse 2: Lazy thing! She's going the right way to get disciplined. (*Making incorrect inference.*)
Nurse 1: But she was ill! (*Retrieving the conversation by elaborating/clarifying.*)

Exercise 3.5 Instruction and attenuated communication

Instructions

1. Divide into pairs. You will each need three rectangular pieces of paper, approximately 20 cm × 10 cm.
2. Sit back to back to your partner. Arrange your pieces of paper on the floor in front of you. Choose as irregular pattern as you like, but make sure that each piece touches another in at least one place.
3. Instruct your partner in how to arrange her/his sheets of paper so that she/he ends up with the paper in the same arrangement. No looking is allowed, although clarification can be asked for.
4. When the pieces of paper are arranged to satisfaction, examine the similarities between the arrangements. Discuss the reasons for any differences.
5. Swop over, and repeat the exercise. This time use as irregular pattern as you can.
6. Discuss the finished arrangements and consider the discussion issues.

Discussion issues

1. What strategies of explanation were used? For example, were analogies drawn, metaphors used, comments about relational aspects made, etc.?
2. Did questioning help clarify the arrangement? Why/why not?
3. Was a different strategy adopted the second time round? If so, how?
4. Would the strategies have been different if you were explaining to an older or younger person? If so, how!
5. Did anybody get frustrated? If so, how did this affect helpful communication?
6. Are there any analogous situations in nursing? (That is where one person has to explain something to another who cannot see, and where one/both partners easily get frustrated.)
7. Were elaborated/restricted codes used? Did they vary with level of frustration?

Comments

So far, we have considered language choice as the *reflection* of the relationship between partners. It can also *create* a set of relationships. If we deliberately talk in such a way that assumes knowledge that we know our partner *does not* have, we create a *superior* relationship. Similarly, if we elaborate our conversation, assuming our partner knows nothing, when we know she/he *does* have some relevant knowledge, we again create a situation of superiority. Very many strategies of speech that we use communicate relative status; even if we do not intend a 'status message' to be given, what we say may be interpreted as one. An opportunity to examine strategies of speech and their effect is given in Exercise 3.6.

The only way we really know how our partner has interpreted what we have said is by the way she/he responds and the consequences that follow for the rest of the interaction, and subsequent interactions, with the same partner. The social functions that language serves, and some of the strategies that we all use every day, are summarized in Table 3.2, and examined in detail in Exercise 3.7.

Interaction context

As we noted above, the only way we can really tell whether or not a particular strategy has fulfilled its function is by looking at the effect of using that strategy. Just to know that a joke was made is not very helpful, unless we know that people laughed. Whilst the intentions of a speaker are important, it is far more helpful to be able to judge the reactions of the listener accurately. Only then will we be able to make any necessary adjustments to our own behaviour — an essential component of the effective use of interpersonal skill. In taking the 'other's' reactions into account we are using what is known as the *interaction context* in order to decide how to act appropriately (usually in order to achieve some social goal). It will often be necessary to look at an interaction over a period of time, in order to judge whether or not a particular strategy was effective or not, because examining speech, comment by comment, will not always tell us. Sometimes we may not even know whether a particular strategy was effective or not until we meet again on another occasion. So, for example, we may not know whether what we hoped would be reassuring was so until we meet again and are in a position to assess our partner's anxiety/concern with the issue; if she/he is still anxious at a later date, we may assume our 'reassuring' strategy has been ineffective. This raises an interesting question of how short or long term our strategies are or should be. There is probably no answer to this! Exercise 3.8 aims to give some direct experience of some of the problems of evaluating the efficacy of interpersonal strategies.

Exercise 3.6   Language codes

Instructions

Please collect a sample of conversation, overheard in a nursing setting. Write the conversation down as soon as possible after hearing it, so you manage to record as many of the figures of speech and so on as you can.

Record the speech, for two people (A and B) say, in the following way:

A (1) ...
B (2) ...
A (3) ... etc.

This represents three utterances. You should try to include twenty utterances if possible.

Make a note of the *situation* (place, other people present, context of the conversation), and of *who the people talking were* (not their names, but rather their roles and relationships with each other, if you know them).

Look carefully at your conversation and consider the discussion issues. If possible, talk about it with a partner who has also done the exercise.

Discussion issues

1. Can you identify the goals each person had for this conversation?
2. Can you identify any jargon, restricted codes, latent/manifest meaning confusion, or any strategy of speech?
3. Can you tell what social effect any of these strategies had?
4. Can you think of any better ways that the people could talk in order to achieve their goals?
5. Were any strategies used in order to negotiate roles?
6. What meaning has been lost by only looking at the transcripts of speech?
7. What was it like listening to, writing down and discussing this conversation?

Comments

Table 3.2 Social functions and strategies of speech

Function	Focus	Strategies	Examples
Communication of relative:	Role	'Oneupmanship'	N. When I last spoke to Professor Brown ...
(a) status	Interpersonal attitudes	Name dropping	P. I broke my arm getting my parachute off.
(b) interest		Distraction	N. Sorry ... You were saying?
		Formality of address	N. Good afternoon, Mrs Robinson *v.* Hiya, pet!
			P. Hello, Doctor!
			Chaplain Let us pray!
Identification as member of social group	Role	Formality of address	N. (*on phone*) Good morning, Doctor, Nurse Burrows here.
	Shared knowledge	Talking 'shop'	N. (*to other N.*) ... and then in the afternoon, they both took her to theatre.
		Using jargon	Sister Nurse, did you say the B.P. for No. 6 was 110 over 90?
		Restricted codes	
Personal identity	Character	Personal anecdotes	P. I always went for a walk after Church on Sundays.
	Interests	Self-disclosure	N. When I were a li'l 'un, I 'ad some braw times wi' me da'.
	Values and attitudes	Lies	N. I think canoeing sounds really interesting.
	Interpersonal attitudes		P. (*to N.*) I had a cat that got run over once, too.
			N. Oh, I hate just sitting quietly and reading.
			P. I need to go to the little boys' room.

Control/manipulation (1)	Interpersonal attitudes	Flattery Tact Compliments	Junior Dr (*to student N.*) You *do* do dressings well! P. No, it didn't hurt as much as it could have. N. Oh, you've washed your hair — it does look nice!
Control/manipulation (2)	Encounter Regulations	Greetings Partings Questioning {closed / open / leading} Encouraging Reflecting	P. Hello, and how are you today after your break? N. It's nice to see you looking so well. 'Bye! P. What do you think of it? N. Mm ... Go on ... N. So you would like more information?
Control/manipulation (3)	Regulation of others' (a) behaviour (b) feelings	Instructions Commands Requests Threats Jibes/jokes Reassurance	N. Take both these pills now! N. Turn over! N. Please will you keep a record of the fluids you take today? P. If you do that again, I'm walking out. N. You look like a chip waiting for its vinegar! N. It's quite normal to feel upset.
Instrumental	Getting or achieving something	Requests Hints	P. Will you let me go to the day room now? P. I'm going to burst any minute.
Rewardingness/interest as interaction partner	Character Interests	Colourful speech Humour	N. (*to other N.*) ... it was so fantastic — the heather was vivid and fragrant and the moss as springy as fresh-cut hay. P. (*to N.*) Another injection? No, I don't mind, they don't call me pop-a-bubble Pete for nothing!

Table 3.2 continued

Category	Function	Type		Example
Representational	Inform others	Give information	N.	Go up the corridor and take the first on the right ...
	Role	Answer requests	N.	It will hurt at the time, but should only last 3–4 hours.
			Dr	It's just a little test to see if the nerves are damaged.
Investigative	To acquire information	Questioning	P.	What does D. & C. stand for?
	To learn		N.	Have you been in hospital before?
	Role			
Expressive	Personal identity	Exclamations	P.	I hate sago!
	Emotional state	Swearing	P.	You stick that bleedin' thing in me again ...
		Terms of endearment	N.	(to child) Come on, lovey ...
Escapism	Role	Blocking	N.	How are you feeling? O.K.?
	Interpersonal attitude	Changing the subject	N.	How soon will you recover? ... What did you have for dinner?
	Personal identity	Joking	P.	I'll say hello to St Peter at the Pearly Gates for you.
		False reassurance	N.	Oh come now, there's no need to worry!
		Leading questions	N.	That didn't hurt, did it?
Non-verbal accompaniment	Behaviour	Promising	N.	I promise I'll come and see you later.
	Acts	Betting	P.	I bet you I'll eat it all today.
Descriptions	Statements about the world	Stating	P.	The floor needs cleaning.
	Personal identity	Reporting	N.	(to Sister) Mrs Perkins had a good night.
	Interpersonal attitudes			

Social functions that are not primarily interpersonal

Regulation of own			
(a) behaviour	Self-control	Self-statements	N. Now, 250 cl dextrose …
(b) feelings	Self-reassurance		P. Pull yourself together, it won't be that bad!
Aesthetics	Literature	Creative speech/writing	E.g. poem written to N. by grateful P.
	Poetry		
	Messages		

Source: Derived in part from W.P. Robinson, *Language and Social Behaviour*, Penguin, Harmondsworth, 1972 and M.A.K. Halliday, *Explorations in the Functions of Language*, Arnold, London, 1973.

Exercise 3.7   Functions and strategies of speech (1)

Instructions

Look at Table 3.2. Try to generate your own examples of different strategies of speech to illustrate each function. If you can, restrict your examples to nursing settings.

If you find any of the functions particularly hard to illustrate, discuss the function with a partner who has also tried to do the exercise.

When you have tried to illustrate every function, consider the Discussion Issues.

Discussion issues

1. Which functions of speech are the most common in nurse–patient interactions? Why do you think this is?
2. Which are the most common functions of speech fulfilled by patients? What factors produce this situation?
3. Do doctor–nurse interactions reveal some functions of speech more than others? Which and why might this be?
4. Are there any functions of speech that are rarely found in nursing settings? Which, and why might this be?

Comments

An important lesson to be drawn from Exercise 3.8 is that *perceptual* aspects of interpersonal skill are just as important as *performance* aspects, if not more so. If we are to monitor the effects of our own behaviour in order to ascertain whether we have been effective or not, and if we are to try to judge our partners' position (feelings, attitudes, etc.) we must develop the skills of interpersonal perception. (see Section 3.3).

Interdependence of non-verbal behaviour and speech

Before we start to consider social and interpersonal perception, it is, perhaps worth reconsidering the interrelations between speech and non-verbal behaviour. Most encounters involve both speech and non-verbal behaviour in complex interaction, and whilst it can be useful to look at the channels separately, we should also try to examine the whole, as in Exercise 3.9.

Whilst we notice both verbal and non-verbal behaviours, and sometimes the interaction between the two, we use many other cues to interpret what we see/hear. Behaviour that means something in one setting will mean something else in another, or between different people, or observed by somebody else. It is very difficult to claim that there is such a thing as veridical (or true) perception of social behaviour. Exercise 3.9 is particularly useful for pointing to the difference between observation and perception which includes interpretation. Even observations are subject to biases due to our personal characteristics and skill (or lack of it). We will go on to discuss some of the factors that influence our perception of social behaviour and other people. If we are to make any sense at all of our own and other people's behaviour, we must be aware of the nature of social perception.

3.3 Social perception

Interpersonal skill is not solely concerned with what we say or do; it is equally concerned with how astute we are in observing what other people say and do, and how we interpret what we notice. This sounds easy: either someone says/does something, or she/he does not. The problem is, though, that most people say and do far too much for us to notice and remember accurately everything that really happened. In fact, in our everyday lives we are extremely selective in what we notice about other people. We make all sorts of judgements about others on the basis of a limited amount of *factual*

Exercise 3.8   Functions and strategies of speech (2)

Instructions

Look at a film of a nursing interaction. Your library may have some video tapes that you can watch. Failing this, watch some television scenes of nurses (if possible, watch documentaries, but feature/soap opera scenes will do).

As you watch the scene, write down your observations of effective and ineffective strategies in the chart below. Repeat, for at least one further nursing interaction.

With another person, if possible one who has also completed the exercise, consider the discussion issues. It is interesting to watch the same scene as a partner, and to compare notes.

Answer sheet

	Interaction I	Interaction II
Strategy (What was said?)		
Outcome (What was the affect?)		
Alternative (Was there a better way to say it?)		
Overall impression		

Discussion issues

1. Did any sequence stand out as an example of particularly good or poor use of interpersonal skill? In what ways was it good or bad?
2. How are judgements about the efficacy of interpersonal skill made?
3. What cues did you use to make your judgements about the overall impression?
4. Did any factors, other than the actors' own abilities directly affect their levels of interpersonal skill? What were they?
5. What problems were there in attempting to take notes whilst watching or reading the interactions?

Comments

---

information. As we grow up, we develop cognitive or mental frameworks that help us organize, interpret and remember the plethora of social information available to us in any situation. These frameworks are known as *schemata*. We form schemata from what we know about ourselves and other people, and from our general experience with life. Once formed, the schemata determine both the ease with which new social information is processed and the efficiency with which it is brought to mind (see Figure 3.2).

Our schemata encourage us to be extremely selective in what we perceive in other people's behaviour. On entering an unfamiliar ward, qualified nurses, student nurses and 'lay' visitors will all perceive very different things about the nurses working on that ward. Their previous experiences have led to the formation of different cognitive frameworks, and different sets of expectations relating to how the nurses will be behaving. So if they all find that some of the nurses are sitting on the beds, smoking, the qualified nurses may be horrified, the student nurses may be bemused but assume this ward permits such things. and the lay visitors may not even notice anything strange. So, whilst our schemata are formed on the basis of past experience, they can lead to distortions or biases in what we perceive. For a start, we only *attend* to certain things and not to others. Often, those things we notice are of particular relevance to us for one reason or another. In the above example, the lay visitors may have been far more interested in detecting the whereabouts of the patients they had come to visit than in the activities of the nurses: nurses, on the other hand, would be particularly interested in nurse behaviour. So what they each notice is of personal relevance.

Sometimes we even make up things that we think are happening but are not: in other words, we *construct* social events. If these events have taken place some time previously, we *reconstruct* social events. In doing this, we remember some things and then assume certain other things (must have) happened as well. Again, taking the above example, the qualified nurses might have been so shocked at what they saw that they perceived *all* the

Exercise 3.9   Observation of social behaviour

Instructions

1. Please make some observations of people in a variety of different social situations. Observe:

   (a) two people together at the same time, but who are not interacting with each other;
   (b) two people interacting together;
   (c) a group of people (more than 3) interacting;
   (d) a group of people (more than 3) interacting, of which you are one.

2. For each observation, note:

   (a) the setting;
   (b) what you saw and heard (that is, what you observed);
   (c) what this meant (that is, how you interpreted what you saw and heard);
   (d) how the setting influenced the behaviour;
   (e) how you felt as an observer.

3. Carry out the observations for about 5–10 minutes each. They can take place anywhere.

4. With at least one other person, if possible one who has also completed the exercise, consider the discussion issues.

Discussion issues

1. Were non-verbal behaviours easier to observe than speech? Why/why not?
2. Were any of the observations particularly problematic? If so, which ones, and why?
3. How important was the setting for your interpretations?
4. On what other bases did you make your interpretations?
5. Did you have any difficulty separating *observation* from *interpretation*? Why?
6. Did your feelings as observer affect your observations at all? If so, how?
7. What are the major problems in observing 'natural' social behaviour? How may these be overcome?

Comments

Figure 3.2   The development and function of schemata in social perception

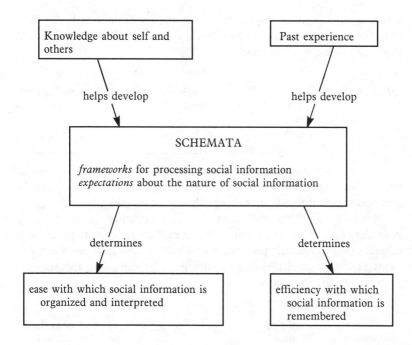

nurses to have been sitting on the beds smoking, when in fact, only some of them were. On relating the incident later, the student nurses, too, on assuming that the 'permissive' regime of the ward enabled some of the nurses to be smoking, may generalize their account to include an observation that 'visitors are allowed at any time', when they have no evidence that this is so.

Many of these biases in person perception are due to the expectations we hold about what should (and what did) happen. These expectations come from various sources, and we will consider some of these now.

Labelling

When we hold expectations about other people's behaviour, attitudes, beliefs, character, etc. by virtue of the role they play, labelling may occur. The labelling process is as follows:

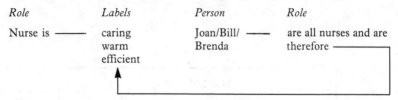

Role	*Labels*	*Person*	*Role*
Nurse is ——	caring warm efficient	Joan/Bill/ —— Brenda	are all nurses and are therefore

We expect that the *person* will possess the characteristics associated with the *role*. If these expectations are widely held, the person becomes 'labelled' and may find it very difficult not to adopt those characteristics.

Take, for example, the staff nurse who has a reputation for being willing to swop duty rotas at the last minute. She/he may get so many requests for last-minute changes, assuming she/he will be willing, that however much she/he wants not to swop, she/he ends up doing so. Exercise 3.10 focuses on this process. The process is as follows:

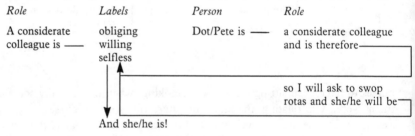

Role	*Labels*	*Person*	*Role*
A considerate colleague is ——	obliging willing selfless	Dot/Pete is ——	a considerate colleague and is therefore
			so I will ask to swop rotas and she/he will be

And she/he is!

Labelling may result in a *self-fulfilling prophecy* (that is if we expect things to happen, they will), and is linked to the existence of stereotypes.

Exercise 3.10   Expectations and labelling

Instructions

When you became the grade of nurse that you are now (first-year student/pupil; third-year student; staff nurse, etc.) did your behaviour change? List the ways your behaviour changed and try to think of the reasons for the changes.

Answer sheet

Changes in behaviour   *Reasons for these changes*

1. Did any of the changes surprise you, in that you would not have expected yourself to have acted like this?
2. Did you have any expectations of how to play your new role? If so, what were they?
3. Did (or does) labelling affect the ways in which other people act and react towards you? If so, how?
4. In your student/professional group, are you cast in an informal role (for example, know-it-all, joker, leader, etc.)? What is it? How has this occurred and what effect does it have on how you behave in the group?
5. When you have thought about and answered the above questions, consider the discussion issues.

Discussion issues

1. Have you seen any examples of labelling in your work as a nurse? Please describe.
2. How do nurses' expectations affect the behaviour of patients?
3. How do patients' own expectations about how they are to behave affect their behaviour when they are ill? Do these expectations have any repercussions for nurses?
4. Where do (a) patients, (b) relatives and (c) nurses get their expectations about each other from?

Comments

Stereotypes

Stereotypes are generalized statements about things. We all use stereotypes to help us organize and understand our social worlds. The process of stereotyping requires us to categorize things, attribute characteristics to the category and then infer that the things, themselves, possess those characteristics by virtue of belonging to the category. We can hold stereotypes about people, objects, cultures, food, roles — anything in fact. Some of this diversity is illustrated in Exercise 3.11.

When we stereotype roles, there is a danger that this can lead to labelling and, in turn, to *self-fulfilling prophecies*. Some of the stereotypes we have are widely held, but others are more idiosyncratic and specific to ourselves. When these are concerned with the 'typical' characteristics different 'types' of people have, they are known as implicit personality theories.

Implicit personality theories

We all have ideas about the ways different types of people behave and why they do so. In other words we all have our own 'theories of personality'. These theories are personal to ourselves and may not be shared by others. They arise primarily from our experiences of other people, our prejudices and our likes/dislikes. However, we may have adopted certain beliefs about others from, for example, our parents: these may then be incorporated into our implicit personality theories. Some examples of implicit personality statements might be: 'People who wear Hush Puppies are mean'; 'Drivers wearing hats are unpredictable'; 'Staff nurses over thirty are pompous'; 'Women who wear red lipstick are reliable'; and so on. We use our implicit theories of personality in order to make predictions (often wrongly) about how people we do not know very well behave, and thus how we should behave in relation to them. Exposure to one's own and others' implicit personality theories is offered in Exercise 3.12.

Our implicit personality theories are particularly important, as we have said above, when first meeting people. They help us form impressions of people which are, generally, hard to change. Having made judgements about people, we tend to regard everything they do in a light that is consistent with our initial judgements. Thus, implicit personality theories, too, may lead to a self-fulfilling prophecy, through our desire to maintain consistency.

Exercise 3.11   Stereotyping

Instructions

Please describe what you think the typical characteristics of people/objects/places are. Distinguish between those you know well, those about which you have some information, and those about which you know little. Use any information that you can, including your own past experience. Do not spend more than 5 minutes on any one thing. Write the typical characteristics of your chosen person/object/place in the chart below.

Answer sheet

1. Well known

2. Some information

3. Little information

   Discuss your answers with a colleague who has also completed the exercise if possible, and consider the discussion issues.

Discussion issues

1. How similar were the typical characteristics of the people/objects/places in the different categories? Why might this be?
2. Where do the ideas you have produced come from?
3. How useful are such stereotypes?
4. Can we do without stereotypes? Why/why not?
5. How likely are stereotypes to lead to the self-fulfilling prophecy?

Comments

Exercise 3.12   Implicit personality theories

Instructions

Please think of the tutor who has taken your last class session. What is she/he like?

Answer sheet

	What is she/he like?	*What led you to make this judgement?*
Age		
Background		
Personality		
Beliefs, values and attitudes		
Interests		
Living style (type of house, marital status, children, diet, etc.)		

With one or two colleagues who have also done the same task, consider the discussion issues.

Discussion issues

1. Was there much agreement? Why/why not?
2. How much was based on 'fact'?
3. Were implicit and/or general stereotypes used?
4. Were any characteristics similar to your own or other peoples'?
5. Have you employed implicit personality theories in your nursing career? When/how?

Comments

Consistency

In many different spheres of our social lives we seem to try to maintain consistency. This is particularly so when we make social judgements. Having once described a ward sister as easy to get on with, it would take a lot of contradictory instances to make us change our minds. Similarly, if we initially experience a porter as aggressive and surly, we will be wary of him/her in the future. Although we like to think that they are not, first impressions are very resistant to change. We distort or explain away contradictory information so that we can uphold the consistency of our initial judgement. Suppose, for example, the sister who is 'easy to get on with' is rude and offhand the next time we meet her: we may well assume she has had a bad day or does not feel too good. Basically, we will still see her as 'easy to get on with'. It has been suggested that we tend to group characteristics together, around the 'central traits' of *warm* and *cold*. Once we have judged people to be 'warm', or to possess some of the characteristics that are grouped around 'warm', we tend not to judge them as 'cold'. And of course, the converse also holds: having judged people to be 'cold', in order to maintain consistency in our judgements, we do not also see them as 'warm'. The extent to which this holds true may be gauged from Exercise 3.13.

Once we have made preliminary judgements about people in terms of their being warm or cold, our subsequent perceptions of them might be distorted as we strive to maintain consistency. A *halo effect* is said to operate. Take for example the instance of a colleague we have judged to be matter-of-fact and unfeeling. With absolutely no 'evidence' to go on, we may also think of her/him as impatient, selfish and argumentative. We generalize our perceptions of her/him from our initial impressions. The danger here, again, is that the operation of the *halo effect* and the maintenance of consistency in judgements about people may lead to a *self-fulfilling prophecy*.

Personal relevance

At the beginning of this section, we mentioned that we are selective in what we notice about other people. What we perceive is influenced by our schemata: by our expectations, our stereotypes, our implicit personality theories and our need to maintain consistency. We will also perceive those things that have *personal significance*, especially those characteristics we can identify with and that we judge to be similar to our own. Thus, when we meet

Exercise 3.13   Central traits and consistency

Instructions

Please list as many characteristics of people as you can, under the heading of each of the two 'central traits'.

Answer sheet

Warm   *Cold*

Consider the discussion issues.

Discussion issues

1. Think of two people you know, one of whom you consider to be *warm* and one *cold*. If you were to describe her/him, would you use traits from both of the lists, above?
2. Could you predict how this person might react to an acquaintance who was upset?
3. How did you make these decisions?
4. How might the issue of '*consistency around central traits*' affect your interpersonal behaviour as a nurse?

Comments

someone who shares our values, attitudes or beliefs, or even a particular interest, we will judge him/her positively and attribute favourable characteristics to him/her. Furthermore, we may even generalize many of our own characteristics to him/her. This is another example of a *halo effect* at work. The distortions in perception that occur will be particularly strong if we share attitudes, values, beliefs and interests with the other person. The distortions are not, however, limited to these areas. The student nurse, far from home, may be overjoyed to find the first patient she/he gets to know comes from her/his home town: the joy is magnified if they both attended the same school, etc. It will take this nurse a long time to recognize she/he dislikes the patient. More crucially, if, for example, the patient reveals some emotional concern, the nurse may 'jump' to an interpretation of what the patient is *really* saying far too quickly — assuming that as they are 'so alike' (but are they?) she/he really understands him/her. In this way a relationship may develop between them that is founded on false assumptions and contains many misperceptions.

Similar biases may emerge if we perceive the person as having characteristics dissimilar to our own. If we are fat, we may note immediately that our new acquaintance is painfully thin; others present for whom fat/thinness is irrelevant may not even notice. As before, selective perception, based on personal relevance, may lead to generalized expectancies and a *self-fulfilling prophecy*. The selectivity of perception is illustrated in Exercise 3.14.

Constructive and reconstructive social perception

We have seen in this section that 'accurate', 'objective' social perception is difficult to achieve. We *construct* our observations and interpretations of interpersonal events on the basis of the schemata we have developed over the years. Our expectations (based on past experience, anticipation of the future and present knowledge) encourage us to make unwarranted generalizations and to try to maintain consistency of judgements. As a result, much of what we 'perceive' to be the case may become a *self-fulfilling prophecy*, and turn out as expected. Similar biases are produced when we *reconstruct* our perceptions, based on (unreliable) memory. We have seen (Exercise 3.14) that eye-witness testimony is notoriously unreliable. So, too, is the evidence of our ears, as shown in Exercise 3.15.

Exercise 3.14   Selective perception

Instructions

With a partner please think of a person you have both seen recently for a short period of time (for example, canteen staff, bus passenger, shop keeper, etc). Answer the following questions about him/her.

Answer sheet

1. Was she/he taller/shorter than 5 ft 2 in (female) 5 ft 8 in (male)?
2. Was her/his hair light/dark?
3. Was she/he fat/thin?
4. Was she/he wearing a cardigan or a jumper?
5. Did she have on make-up?
6. Did he have a beard?
7. What colour was her/his shirt?
8. Was she/he wearing glasses?
9. Did she/he have light/dark trousers (or skirt)?
10. Was she/he wearing a belt?
11. Was she/he carrying a notepad or case?
12. Did she/he or other people speak the most?
13. Did she/he smile?
14. Did she/he say 'please' or 'thank you'?
15. Did you like her/him? (Why/Why not?)
16. How long did she/he stay?
17. What questions did she/he ask?

Discuss with each other your answers with reference to the discussion issues.

Discussion issues

1. How similar were the answers?
2. Do any of your answers depend on you? (For example, how fat/thin you are etc?)
3. Do any of the answers depend on the person's role?
4. If there were differences in the answers what does this say about the reality of social perception?

Comments

Exercise 3.15   Reconstruction of memory

For this exercise you will need to be in groups of between 6 and 15 people.

Instructions

One person in the group read one of the messages as shown on page 332. Read it through once then tell the next person what the message is. That person should tell the next person what the message was and so on until everybody has been told the message. The last person to receive the message should write the message down. Repeat this with reference to all the messages on page 332 and giving the messages in a different order throughout the group. When all the messages have been given, discuss the differences between the real message as shown on page 332 and the last message that the last person in the group has written down. Discuss the exercise with reference to the discussion issues.

Discussion issues

1. How did distortions in the message occur?
2. What aspects of the message were retained/excluded?
3. How can nurses ensure that (a) they do not reconstruct messages, and (b) that they give information in such a way as to reduce the likelihood that others will reconstruct what they have heard?

Comments

Figure 3.3   Social perception and the self-fulfilling prophecy

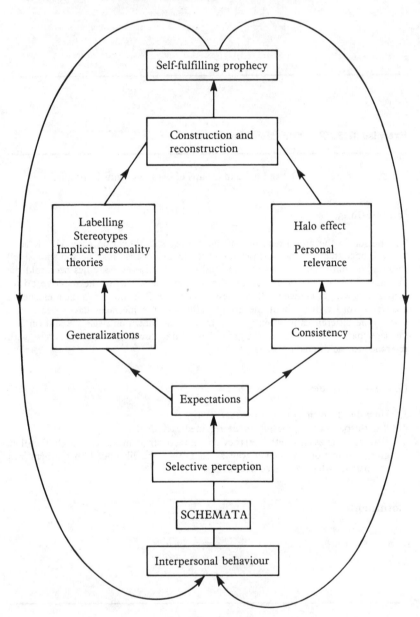

Our predisposition to construct and/or reconstruct our perceptions of other people can have serious consequences for our effective use of interpersonal skills in nursing. Perhaps the most crucial effect of the biases inherent in person perception is that they obscure us to the very *individual* nature of the other people we relate to. We are, in effect, 'blinded' to what other people are really doing and saying; this in turn may lead to the adoption of those behaviours, expressions of feelings, etc. that we have *expected*. In other words the *self-fulfilling prophecy* is realized, and we thereafter assume our initial perceptions were accurate! The process is illustrated in Figure 3.3.

It is important for us to bear in mind some of the sources of bias in person perception, and what our own tendencies to be consistent and/or to generalize are, if we are to begin to be able to make realistic observations, assessments and appraisals of our own interpersonal behaviour.

3.4 Summary

This chapter has been concerned with verbal and non-verbal elements of social behaviour and the biases that underlie social perception. Specifically the following issues were raised:

Non-verbal communication and speech interrelate in complex ways.

Non-verbal cues form the bases of impressions of other peoples' values, attitudes, personality and interests.

The meaning of social behaviour is linked to expectations stemming from the cultural and situational context in which it occurred.

Habits are learnt, convey little meaning and are difficult to change.

Non-verbal communication is vital to the regulation of encounters.

Dominance is achieved through the use of certain non-verbal behaviours.

There are latent and manifest meanings in speech.

Rules of conversation vary with culture and situation.

Breaking rules of conversation may be meaningful.

The context contributes to understanding of conversations.

Regular patterns of speech, bound by rules, are called rituals.

Rituals of speech occur in both formal and informal situations.

Strategies of speech vary with role.

Elaborated and restricted styles of speech have different social consequences.

Language style both reflects and creates social relationships.

The value of particular strategies of speech may be assessed from social reactions to them.

Interaction contexts dictate which strategies of speech will be most effective.

Perceptual aspects of interpersonal skill are as important as performance aspects.

Observations about other people are selective, and interpretations of observations open to distortion.

Schemata, or cognitive frameworks, develop that help us organize, interpret and remember social information.

Schemata develop from our knowledge of self and others, and from past experience.

Schemata lead us to be selective in our perceptions and to hold expectations about what is happening.

Expectations lead to the construction and reconstruction of social events.

Expectations are the source of many different biases in social perception.

Labelling may occur when expectations are held by virtue of another's role.

Stereotyping may occur when expectations are held by virtue of categories of attributes.

Expectations based on past experience may lead to the development of implicit personality theories.

Most people attempt to maintain consistency between social judgements.

First impressions are difficult to change, and may lead to a halo effect.

Initial judgements about others frequently include either 'warm' or 'cold', which are thought to be central traits.

Social judgements are often made on the basis of personal relevance.

Expectations lead to the construction and reconstruction of social events, and this in turn may lead to the self-fulfilling prophecy.

The self-fulfilling prophecy may lead to behaviours, or expressions of feelings, resulting from underlying expectations rather than from the person him/herself.

Biases in social perception mitigate against one person treating another as an *individual*, and thus distort the effective use of interpersonal skills.

Further reading

Argyle, M. (1982) Verbal and non-verbal communication (ch. 2), Perception of others (ch. 5), *The Psychology of Interpersonal Behaviour* (4th ed), Penguin, Harmondsworth

Argyle, M. and Trower, P. (1979) The two languages of humans (ch. 2), Judging other people (ch. 3), *Person to Person: Ways of Communicating*, Harper and Row, London

Gahagan, J. (1984) Communication, language and social interaction (ch. 4), Non-verbal communication (ch. 5), *Social Interaction and Its Management*, Methuen, London

Macleod Clark, J. (1984) Verbal communication in nursing. In A. Faulkner (Ed.) *Recent Advances in Nursing, 7, Communication*, Churchill Livingstone, Edinburgh

Stockwell, F. (1972) *The Unpopular Patient*, R.C.N., London (reprinted Croom Helm, London, 1984)

Strongman, K.T. (1979) Judgements and impressions of personality (ch. 13), *Psychology for the Paramedical Professions*, Croom Helm, London

CHAPTER 4

SOCIAL ROUTINES

A great deal of social behaviour is predictable, following regular patterns. We saw in section 3.2 that the concept of 'ritual' is useful to describe regular patterns of speech, based on a shared understanding of its meaning by both speaker and listener. The notion of social ritual, however, extends beyond speech to encompass regular patterns of complex social behaviour. In this section we shall examine the extent to which such patterns of behaviour are linked to the roles that people occupy and the rules they follow.

4.1 Social roles

The concept of 'role' stems from an idea that life is like the theatre: just as actors play different parts in different plays, each with its appropriate scenery, props and scripts, so people occupy roles in different situations, each with its setting, props and expectations held by all the people involved. Roles are, then, the parts we play or the behaviours that are expected from people who occupy different positions in different situations. The more formal the role, the fewer are the variations in behaviour associated with that role. Various pressures are brought to bear on people enacting their roles.

Firstly, the situation itself makes different demands on people occupying different positions. So the ward situation *demands* different behaviour from student nurses, ward sister, consultant, patients, visitors, etc. Sometimes these demands are made explicit (for example, 'No visitors to enter the ward until the screen is removed'), but sometimes they are implicit (for example, patients should not wander about while a ward round is in progress). The less clearly stated the demand, the more scope there is for people to express their role in their own fashion, but also the more likelihood they will make 'mistakes' and behave inappropriately. Secondly, the *expectations* we and others have regarding how those in given positions *should* behave, create pressures to learn appropriate behaviour. The stronger these expectations — or the stronger we believe them to be — the greater the pressures. If, for example, the ward sister expects her nurses to chat to patients, they will; if she does not, they are unlikely to. Again, the more explicit the expectations, the less likelihood that inappropriate behaviour will develop. The third influence is that wielded by the role partner: in order to give meaning to a role, there must be a complementary role. So for the role of 'nurse' to be meaningful, there must be patients/doctors/social workers, and so on. The ways our role partners act towards us, and expect us to behave, help us behave appropriately in our role. Thus we can see that roles are defined and constrainted by (sets of) *expectations*.

Role conflict

Whenever there is conflict between one (set of) expectation(s) and another, we experience role conflict, and this can have repercussions for both how we behave and how we feel. Examples of role strain/conflict are shown in Figure 4.1, and explored in Exercise 4.1.

Whenever we experience role conflict or strain, we try to resolve it in some way in order to reduce it. The social system, itself, often provides a means of coming to terms with the competing expectations of role partners and the demands of new situations. The period of training for nurses is an example of 'easing' people into a new role so they learn how to cope with all the expectations that are placed on them. 'Student nurse' is an interesting example, as the 'easing-in' period is often missed, because the students are placed quickly in positions of responsibility. This situation is made more difficult as one of the most significant role partners — patients — often expect the student nurses on their first day on the ward to know everything and be totally competent. They do not always distinguish between 'student nurse' and 'nurse'. As patients express their expectations regarding knowledge and competence, students may feel a lot of pressure to present themselves in a

Figure 4.1   Role strain

1. Different expectations or lack of agreement amongst role partners

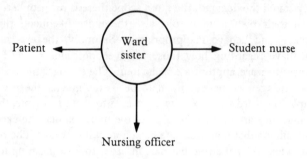

2. Different expectations or lack of agreement between role partners

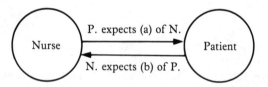

3. Personal expectations differ from situational demands

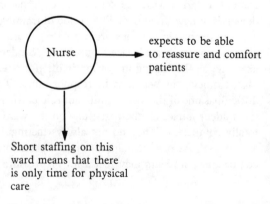

4. Expectations from role partners clash with own principles

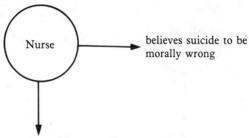

5. Lack of clarity in situational demands

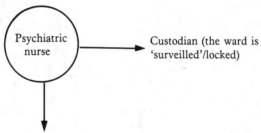

6. Personal characteristics unable to fulfil expectations

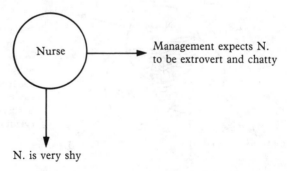

Figure 4.1 continued

7.   Multiple occupancy

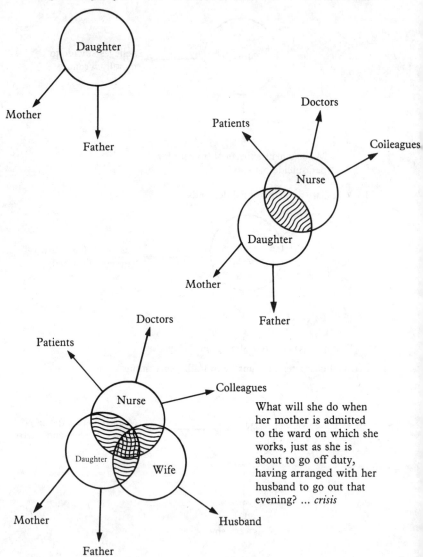

What will she do when her mother is admitted to the ward on which she works, just as she is about to go off duty, having arranged with her husband to go out that evening? ... *crisis*

Exercise 4.1   Role strain

Instructions

Make sure you are familiar with the concept of role strain. Think of yourself, and try to complete each of the following diagrams illustrating different sources of role strain. Note possible ways of resolving the role strain in each case. Use Figure 4.1 as an example if you are not clear about the differences between various sources of strain.

Answer sheet

Sources of role strain and its resolution

1. Different expectations or lack of agreement amongst role partners

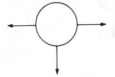

Resolution:

2. Different expectations or lack of agreement between role partners

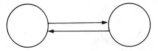

Resolution:

3. Personal expectations differ from situational demands

Resolution:

4.   Expectations from role partners clash with own principles

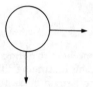

Resolution:

5.   Lack of clarity in situational demands

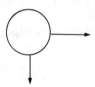

Resolution:

6.   Personal characteristics unable to fulfil expectations

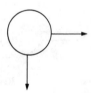

Resolution:

7. Multiple occupancy

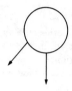

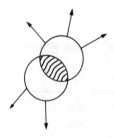

Crisis situation:

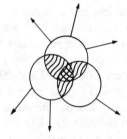

Resolution:

With one or two other people who have also completed the exercise if possible, consider the discussion issues.

Discussion issues

1. Were some sources of role strain easier to identify than others? Why?
2. Are there common ways of resolving role strain? What are they?
3. How easy is it to 'escape' from other people's expectations?
4. Can 'role' and role expectation account for all interaction behaviour? If not, what are the shortcomings of such an analysis?

Comments:

knowledgeable and competent way, when they might really be feeling quite insecure and unconfident. Nevertheless, the period as a student does allow nurses to learn the appropriate 'nurse' behaviours.

When we experience conflict through multiple role occupancy, the easiest way to resolve it, is to prioritize roles. So the nurse who is a single parent might prioritize the 'father' role, rather than the 'nurse' role, when his child is sick. Similarly the newly promoted ward sister may prioritize the role of 'sister' rather than 'friend' when a crisis occurs on her ward and she has to be more firm with her erstwhile friends/colleagues. A further method we have of resolving role conflict is to take some personal action. The nurse who feels conflict at being asked to do something she/he morally disagrees with may either rationalize her/his situation ('I'm sure it won't matter, just this once') or may opt out of the strained role altogether ('If this is what I'm expected to do as a nurse, it's not for me — I'm leaving'). There is quite a bit of evidence to suggest that one of the reasons why student nurses leave the profession is because of the conflict they experience between the reality of the demands made on them as nurses, and what they perceive the public's expectations of them as nurses to be.

We have seen that roles are defined by sets of expectations that we, and others, have of the appropriate behaviours associated with them. These expectations may lead to the experience of role strain or conflict which we try to resolve in various ways. The expectations, themselves, come from ourselves as individuals, the groups to which we belong, the organizations in which we work or even from the wider social/cultural context in which we live. They are transmitted by norms or social rules, which we learn via the process of *socialization*.

4.2 Norms and social rules

Norms and social rules influence both the expression of roles and the expectations surrounding them. Given a particular role, the norms or rules give some guidance as to how it should be expressed. Thus roles and rules are closely linked, and together form what is known as the role-rule context of interpersonal behaviour.

In Exercise 4.2 people's behaviour will have been affected by the extent to which they feel an important part of the class group or identified with the role of 'class member'. The exercise will have evoked, for some people, thoughts such as 'I am a member of this group; we did not do well; I must do better ...'. This is the expression of a norm, that is 'I must not let the group down.' The norm itself could have come from the wider social context (for example, 'We should always do our best'), whether this be family, religion, or culture: on the other hand it could have been generated by the group itself as a result of the quality of interaction and relationships that exist. The more cohesive the group, the more individual group members will identify with the group. We cannot examine inter-group relations in any detail here, but feel it is important to introduce the concepts of norms and social rules for several reasons.

First, and perhaps most importantly, the efficacy of interpersonal skills is inextricably linked to role-rule contexts. The acquisition of good interpersonal skill necessitates an appreciation of the nature of different role-rule systems, in order to know *how* to behave and how to interpret other people's behaviour. Furthermore, once we understand the extent to which role-rule systems define and constrain our interactions, we can begin to see that the use of good interpersonal skills is not only restricted by the people displaying those skills, but is in part determined by the culture, the situation and other people's expectations. In other words, interpersonal skill is not to be seen in isolation from the social system: it is, instead, just one facet of interpersonal behaviour and is subject to many other influences. (This theme will be

Exercise 4.2   Group identification

Instructions

Take a sheet of newspaper. Look through the newsprint to identify all letters that have an angle in them. For example, *k, v, w, y,* etc. When you have become familiar with those letters make sure you have a watch with a second hand or a stop-watch. Read backwards through a piece of the newspaper and cross off all those letters that have an angle in them. Do this for one minute exactly. When you have completed the task turn to page 333 for the number of letters that most people are able to find in a piece of newsprint in one minute. If your average falls short of this average total, repeat the exercise. When completed consider the discussion issues that are raised. If possible discuss the exercise with a colleague who has also completed it.

Comments

---

developed further in Chapter 9.) We saw (section 3.3) that strong expectations can result in self-fulfilling prophecies, whereby people may adopt those behaviours expected of them.

Second, the identification of those specific norms that individuals and/or groups adhere to may help us to understand some of the (sub)cultural variations in social behaviour, and adjust our own perceptions and/or behaviour accordingly.

Third, the recognition that norms exist may help us understand some of the regular patterns of behaviour that are associated with both roles and situations. Furthermore, the consequences of either not behaving according to norms, or deliberately breaking the rules are often in terms of the effects this has on interpersonal skills and relationships.

4.3 Social ritual

Social rules form the basis of the regular patterns of behaviours that occur in interpersonal situations, and that vary with role. Two of the most pervasive social rituals are interaction openings and closures.

Openings and closures are of special significance because of their potential for impact on the quality of the encounter: if we 'get off on the wrong foot' the entire interaction may be counter-productive, and if we 'end on a sour note', further interactions may be jeopardized. Generally, openings and closures are highly structured, containing large elements of ritualized behaviours, and are common to many different (sub)cultures.

Interaction openings

The tone of an interaction is usually set by the way it is opened. An opening involves far more than just the words that are spoken. All the non-verbal cues expressed by each person help to give the others an idea about what is to follow. The nurse who approaches the patient slowly, looking down, when she/he is about to give him/her some test results, creates an expectation in the patient about what she/he is about to say. The patient then prepares him/herself for bad news, and might be somewhat bemused if the nurse then gaily tells him/her that the results are fine.

The physical setting of an encounter may also lead people to have expectations about what is to ensue. A patient who finds floor cushions rather than chairs in the clinic when she/he attends as an orthopaedic outpatient, may behave (and expect others to behave) in an unusual fashion.

What is actually said in greeting, or in opening the conversation, is of crucial importance, and tells each participant a great deal about how the other perceives their relationship and expects the interaction to proceed. For the more task-related interactions, the opening may include an attempt by one (or even both) partner to discover the extent to which the other knows about the task to be undertaken. So, on introducing a new topic, a nurse tutor may investigate whether any of the students have studied the area beforehand, prior to launching into it. Similarly, a nurse explaining to a pregnant woman about amniocentesis may first try to discover the extent of the woman's knowledge, so she/he knows how and what to explain about the process and possible side effects. Broadly, the functions of interaction openings are as shown in Table 4.1. How could each of these functions be fulfilled? Many opening sequences serve several functions at once.

Table 4.1   Functions of interaction openings

Social functions	Task or cognitive functions
Attracting and gaining attention	Ascertaining the extent of knowledge held about the topic or the purpose of the encounter
Expressing relationships/roles	
Establishing rapport	Indicating the objectives of the encounter
Arousing the motivation/interest of a partner	
Ascertaining others' expectations	Explaining one's functions and limitations
Indicating the purpose of the encounter	
Establishing links with previous encounters	

Exercise 4.3   Interaction openings

Instructions

Please describe as fully as you can appropriate interaction openings for the following interactions. With reference to Table 4.1 note which functions they fulfil.

Answer sheet

1. You are a student nurse on her/his first day on the ward and are asked to admit a new patient who is sitting in the corridor. You go to speak to her.

    Functions:

2. A parent is visiting a six-year-old child who has slept little the night before. You want to speak to the parent before she/he visits.

    Functions:

3. A middle-aged male patient who has had surgery is to have his sutures removed. You, a nurse, approach him. He appears to be reading a book intently.

Functions:

4. You are on night duty on the children's ward. A little girl of eight years of age is lying awake. You go to speak to her.

Functions:

5. An elderly female patient is weeping silently. You are a nurse. You are passing her bed and stop to speak to her.

Functions:

With a partner who has also completed the exercise, if possible, consider the discussion issues.

Discussion issues

1. What is the relative importance of physical setting, non-verbal behaviour and speech for effective interaction openings?
2. To what extent do the role/rule contexts determine interaction openings?
3. How easy is it to 'recover' misunderstood interaction openings?

Comments

Consider the following:

> *Staff nurse*, in busy accident and emergency unit, receiving young woman with an asthmatic collapse. Her companion is able to give information, but the patient herself is unable to speak. Patient has been brought by ambulance and is propped up on a bed.
>
> N. approaches P., smiling, and puts one hand on her shoulder and the other on her arm. 'Hello Ann, I'm the staff nurse on the ward. You're having a lot of difficulty breathing, I can see. Don't worry, we'll soon have you comfortable. I can't actually give you anything but the doctor will be here soon. He'll give you an injection and probably put up a drip. Have you had a drip before? (*Pause. Waits for non-verbal sign.*) I thought so — so you'll know what to expect.'

Which functions does this opening serve? Other opportunities to consider different interaction openings are given in Exercise 4.3.

Interaction closures

Our feelings of satisfaction with an encounter, liking for our partners, sense of achievement and expectations for future meeting are affected by the way the interaction is closed. As with openings, closures involve both non-verbal and verbal behaviours. Closures can include sequences or episodes of behaviours, and need not be restricted to relatively short parting statements. Different situations require different styles of closure. When a lot of information has been exchanged, closures may be used by either party to summarize or clarify the material that has been covered. If the encounter was highly emotional, as for example in a counselling interaction, closure may be used to 'wind down' and ensure that the distressed person has dealt with, and hopefully dissipated, her/his emotionality. In such circumstances, closure can take quite a lot of the total time devoted to the encounter. If either person is left feeling dissatisfied in any way at the end of the interaction, this can severely affect how she/he approaches future meetings. It is important, therefore, to have a clear idea of *how* we want to leave the interaction, and to possess the skills to put this into practice. A patient may well feel belittled if, after a pleasant and informal conversation with the staff nurse, she/he ends the interaction without giving the patient the opportunity to ask her/him anything about her/his views. Similarly, by suddenly announcing that it's time to go off duty, the nurse may make the patient feel a nuisance: he/she may then be reluctant to engage that nurse in conversation in the future.

Table 4.2 Functions of interaction closures

Social functions	Task or cognitive functions
Encouraging a sense of achievement	Indicating topic is completed (for the moment)
Indicating each other's degree of satisfaction and enjoyment	Focusing attention on essential material covered
Maintaining interest for future encounters	Assisting in consolidating facts, skills, concepts, arguments
Dissipating any agitation that had been aroused	Ascertaining whether the objectives of the encounter have been fulfilled
Communicating interpersonal attitudes	Indicating future courses of action
Indicating nature of future encounters	
Establishing the possibility that rapport is likely in the future	
Terminating attention	

The functions that interaction closure serves are shown in Table 4.2. How could each of these functions be fulfilled? Some of the strategies that can be used in closures are similar to those used in openings. The use of open questions can ascertain whether any information reported has been absorbed, or whether our partner has some 'unfinished business' (usually of an emotional nature) that should be dealt with.

If we want to leave the situation in a positive way, we should generally try to end on a supportive note. So, for example, a patient who has just cooperated with a painful procedure, such as a lumbar puncture, may be told 'You did very well, there. It's not easy having that done. You really were helpful,' in a convincing way. These task-related comments may then be followed by some socially supportive comment, such as, 'How do you feel now it's over?.' This will only be valuable if full attention is paid to the reply, and the question is not asked in an accusing way that is really saying, 'Don't you dare say anything other than "O.K."!' It is interesting that when we end informal (rather than task-related) encounters, we often do so by making an excuse, such as, 'Ah well, I must go and see to Mrs Brown now ...,' rather than by saying something socially supportive, such as, 'I've enjoyed our talk — I'll be on duty tomorrow and perhaps we can have another.' If one of the

Exercise 4.4   Interaction closures

Instructions

Please describe as fully as you can appropriate interaction closures for the following interactions. With reference to Table 4.2 note which functions they fulfil.

Answer sheet

1. You have just completed the history sheet of a patient you had admitted. He is an elderly gentleman who has been explaining how he has been having a great deal of abdominal pain. You need to leave him to go and admit another patient.

   Functions:

2. You have attempted to give a young patient some nasty-tasting medicine, and even after much persuasion she has refused to take it. You feel you cannot spare her any more time, so you decide to leave her without her having taken it. What might you say to her?

   Functions:

3. You have been removing the sutures from the wound of a lady who has had a mastectomy. You have been trying to persuade her to look at the wound but she feels unable to do so. You decide to make her comfortable and leave her. What might you say?

   Functions:

4. You have been giving an injection of intramuscular iron to a young male patient of about 18 years of age. What might you say to him before you leave?

   Functions:

   With a partner who has also completed the exercise if possible, consider the discussion issues.

Discussion issues

1. What is the relative importance of physical setting, non-verbal behaviour and speech for effective interaction closures?
2. To what extent do the role/rule contexts determine interaction closures?
3. How easy is it to 'recover' misunderstood interaction closures?

Comments

functions of closure is to set the scene for our next meeting, the latter strategy will be more effective than the former.

As with openings, closures will usually fulfil more than one function at a time. Consider the following:

Sister (terminating discussion with patient on discharge following neurosurgery): 'Now can we just check those details again. How often must you take the yellow pills? (*Awaits reply.*) Yes, that's right. And do you remember what you must do if you get a dizzy spell? (*Awaits reply.*) Good. And as I said, we'll be writing to your G.P. and we'll be contacting you in the next week or so. So, all being well, we'll not be seeing you again. The outpatients clinic is very friendly though. I'm sure you'll get on O.K. Well, we've enjoyed having you on the ward, and we're all so pleased you've made such good progress. We wish you all the best ... Bye.'

Other opportunities to consider different interaction closures are given in Exercise 4.4.

4.4   Functions of social routines

Interaction openings and closures are examples of ritualized social routines. They vary with the situation, the role of the participants and wider social cultural factors, such as the nationality, age, sex and social class of the participants. Different (sub)cultures and situations have different rules associated with them that prescribe appropriate behaviours. Nevertheless, such routines and rituals help us know how to behave and how to interpret other people's behaviour.

What we must remember is that our own behaviour, too, is likely to be interpreted according to other people's appreciation of the nature of social rules. This may result in a breakdown in social relations that we had not anticipated. The other important thing to note is that interpersonal skill (or lack of it) does not simply reside in ourselves, as individuals. Much of our behaviour is constrained by what is *expected* of us in fulfilling our roles in particular situations. We must be aware of this if we are to plan *effective* use of interpersonal skills. In subsequent sections we will explore these underlying issues in greater detail and in relation to more complex interactions.

4.5 Summary

This section has been concerned with the nature of social roles, rules and routines or rituals, taking interaction openings and closures as examples. Specifically, the following issues were raised:

Sequences or episodes of interactions often follow regular patterns.

These patterns of behaviour are linked to the role-rule context in which they occur.

Roles are defined by (sets of) expectations.

Role expectations derive from the (sub)culture, the situation, and other people.

Role conflict or strain occurs as a consequence of different sets of expectations.

Role conflict or strain usually results in an attempt to reduce/resolve the discomfort.

Socialization is the means whereby we learn the rules associated with particular roles.

Social rules or norms derive from the wider social/cultural context or from within groups.

Social rules or norms underlie patterns or rituals in social behaviour.

Two examples of highly structured, ritualized routines are interaction openings and closures.

Opening and closure episodes consist of verbal and non-verbal elements and vary in their length and complexity.

Social and task/cognitive functions can be identified for both openings and closures.

Social rituals vary with the role-rule context.

People from similar (sub)cultures share an understanding of important social rituals.

Breakdown in social relations may occur as a result of misunderstandings of social rituals.

Interpersonal skill does not reside solely in the individual, but is, instead, a product of the role-rule context.

Further reading

French, P. (1983) Communication skills, *Social Skills and Nursing Practice*, Croom Helm, London, Ch. 2

Goffman, E. (1971) *Relations in Public: Microstudies of the Public Order*, Penguin, Harmondsworth

Hargie, O., Saunders, C. and Dickson, D. (1981) Set induction and set closure, *Social Skills in Interpersonal Communication*, Croom Helm, London, Ch. 6

Kagan, C. (Ed.) (1985) The context of interpersonal skills in nursing, *Interpersonal Skills in Nursing: Research and Applications*, Croom Helm, London, Part 2

Murray, M. (1983) Role conflict and intention to leave nursing, *Journal of Advanced Nursing*, Vol. 8, pp 29–31

Roch, J. (1980) The use and limitations of the concept of role for nurse education, *Nursing Times*, 8 May, pp 837–41

CHAPTER 5

FACILITATION AND THE DEVELOPMENT OF RAPPORT

One of the most important things about our interactions with each other, is the extent to which we enjoy them. When we come to examine just what it is that makes an interaction enjoyable, we can usually point out that it has been rewarding in some way, that is we have 'got something out of it'. Generally, we only form relationships with other people on a friendly basis if the rewards of doing so outweigh the costs. The more rewards there are, the stronger the relationship will be, and it is reward or satisfaction that keeps the relationship going. It is rather different if we have a role relationship with someone, such as sister– staff nurse, nurse–patient, and so on, as we will find there are often task-related activities associated with the role that force us to interact.

However, not all the encounters we have in our different roles are connected to tasks. We may simply be chatting to pass the time, keeping each other company, reassuring each other, explaining things to each other, or getting to know each other on an informal basis; this is particularly true of many nursing interactions. For these casual encounters, and for those that are related to the emotional needs of one or other of the interactants, we know that we need to be able to 'develop a rapport' with our partner. Unless we do this, we are likely to find that our relationships are unsatisfying, not at all enjoyable and superficial. But what exactly does it mean, 'to develop a rapport', and how do we do it?

5.1 Rapport

In order to develop a rapport, we must be able to pick up all the cues (verbal and non-verbal) that tell us something about our partners' inner feelings or emotions, and their attitudes towards themselves, us and the situation they are in. Moreover, we must be able to let our partners know that we have picked up these signals, that we understand them, and as far as possible that we will try to meet any needs they have expressed. So, if we notice, for example, that someone is indicating that she/he is afraid, we must try and reassure her/him and so on. If we misunderstand and/or are insensitive, no rapport will be developed and the encounter will not be satisfying to either partner.

Facilitation skills are the ones we use to make interactions rewarding and to develop and maintain rapport. They are not easy skills to use effectively, and misunderstandings will often occur. Even if we are quite good at using these skills in some situations, there will be others where we are not so adept.

In this chapter, we are going to look at some of the issues relating to what we can do to make conversations interesting, how we pick up cues to emotion and interpersonal attitudes, and the specific value of self-disclosure.

5.2 The recognition and expression of emotions

Our ability to develop a rapport depends on whether we can accurately recognize other peoples' inner feelings or emotional states, whether we can communicate this recognition, and whether we can accurately express our own inner feelings appropriately.

The way we recognize others' internal states is to listen to what they say, and, more importantly, to watch what they do. So, whilst people may well say how they are feeling, we often look to the non-verbal cues to get information of how they are *really* feeling. When we talk about emotion, it is useful to think in terms of the six general emotions, and the umpteen other, more specific emotions which are generally considered to be combinations of the six. Table 5.1 gives a rough guide to this way of categorizing emotion.

Different non-verbal cues (or combinations of cues) are associated with different emotions, though we probably rely on the face and the voice for most information. The facial cues that we associate with each emotional state are shown in Exercise 5.1, although it is important to note that we rarely see a facial expression that is stationary. We may well be able to think of patients

Table 5.1   General and specific emotions

Angry	Happy	Sad	Afraid	Disgusted	Surprised/ Interested
Annoyed	Pleased	Sorry	Anxious	Shocked	Amazed
Enraged	Satisfied	Hurt	Alarmed	Sickened	Curious
Irritated	Relieved	Disappointed	Worried	Contemptuous	fascinated
Frustrated	Thrilled	Regretful	Confused		Intrigued

Exercise 5.1   The interpretation of facial and vocal cues of emotion

Instructions

Please look at the combinations of facial and vocal cues given in the chart below. From the box at the side of the chart, choose the appropriate feeling and write in the space provided.

Answer sheet

Facial cues			Feeling	Feelings or Emotions
Brow region	Eye region	Mouth region		
Brows raised	Eyes wide open	Mouth open relaxed		Anger
				Fear
Brows drawn together and raised	Eyes wide	Mouth corners drawn back		Happy
				Disgust
				Sad
Brows lowered, 'knotted'	Eyes wide	Lips pressed or 'squared'		Interest or surprise
Brows lowered	Nose 'screwed up'	Upper lip curled		
Brows lowered at corners	Eyes lowered	Mouth corners down		

Neutral	'Bagging' under eyes, Crows feet, Creases	Mouth corners up

Vocal cues	Feeling
Soft, low, slow, falling inflection, slurred	
Fairly loud, fairly high, rising inflection, fast, variable	
High, varied pitch, fast, rising inflection	
Varied volume, varied pitch, rising inflection	
Loud, high, harsh, clipped, rising and falling inflection	
Slow, slurred	

Source: Adapted from P. Trower, B. Bryant and M. Argyle, *Social Skills and Mental Health*, Methuen, London, 1978

Consider your answers with reference to the discussion issues.

Discussion issues

1. How useful is it to consider stationary expressions?
2. Do some people have permanent, fixed expressions on their faces? Give examples.
3. Would the same cues mean the same if they were used by people of different ages? Please explain.
4. Does the same emotional expression mean something different in different situations (for example, at a pop concert, hospital, funeral, etc.)?
5. What difficulties were there in doing this exercise?

Comments

we would say had 'permanently startled' expressions on their faces: we would still be able to tell when they became anxious. Similarly, we know perfectly well when the nursing officer who 'always wears a frown' is angry. It is the *change* in expression we respond to, not the expression itself.

Other non-verbal cues serve to increase the strength of a feeling expressed. Thus, we know angry people are angrier if they wave their arms about and stamp their feet, but depressed people are more depressed if they keep their arms and legs very still. The non-verbal behaviours that accompany facial and vocal aspects of emotion are called modifiers, as they *modify* the central emotion. Exercise 5.2 focuses on the expression of emotion.

Meaning

In western society, a great deal is made of the need to control our emotions, and nursing is, perhaps, one job where there is even more pressure to do so. What this really means is that we are expected to control the *expression* of emotion, and it is interesting to note that we are, on the whole, very good at controlling our facial and vocal cues. We still give ourselves away, though, by not paying attention to certain other non-verbal cues that then 'leak' contradictory messages. When we wring our hands or wriggle our feet, people may think we are worried, upset or angry. Similarly, if we see someone who appears to be calm, but is scratching her/himself, twiddling her/his hair or chewing her/his fingers we may think she/he is really quite anxious 'underneath'. The cues that 'leak' anxiety are often called self-adaptors, as they are mannerisms that people use in contact with themselves in various ways. We can all think of lots of situations in hospitals where people desperately try to cover up their feelings, but interestingly, they rarely try to hide feelings of joy. In some situations, though, however happy we feel, we may not want to show it. The nurse who gets the job that she/he and her/his friends applied for will not show her/his elation in front of the others: the community nurse who is thrilled to be going on holiday will not let the patient who will miss her/his company know this.

When we think we know the 'real' feeling someone is expressing, because we have picked up certain non-verbal cues, despite her/his attempts to control them, there is the danger that we are wrong. We may be picking up cues that do not, in fact, mean anything. For instance, we may think the new sister is nervous when we notice her biting her nails, but if we then discover that she has bitten her nails all her life, we may change our mind. However, if we see a

Exercise 5.2   The expression and recognition of emotion

Instructions

1. With a partner, allocate the roles A and B.
2. A — Choose one of the general emotions, as shown on the chart. By counting up to 25, communicate that emotion to your partner, getting more and more intense as you count. .
3. B — Identify the emotion that your partner is expressing. Write down on the chart the cues that lead you to make this interpretation.
4. Repeat for all the general emotions.
5. Discuss with each other the signals that A emitted, and any discrepancies between those A intended and that B picked up. Complete the chart together if necessary.

Answer sheet

Counting/contradictory messages

Feeling	Facial cues			Vocal cues	Cues to strength of feeling	Other (such as words used)
	Brows	Eyes	Mouth			
Angry						
Happy						
Sad						
Afraid						
Disgusted						
Interested /surprised						

Comments:

Instructions

1. Swop roles. B is now to express an emotion, and A is now to recognize it, in accordance with the following instructions.
2. B — Please read a sentence communicating a feeling *other* than that indicated by the words in the sentence. See page 333 for examples of sentences. The feeling to be expressed is in brackets at the end of each sentence.
3. A — Identify the emotions being expressed by your partner. Write down the cues that lead you to make this interpretation on the chart.
4. Repeat the exercise communicating feelings that are consistent with the verbal message. Discuss with each other the signals that B emitted, and any discrepancies between B those intended and that A picked up. Complete the chart together if necessary.

Answer sheet

Feeling	Facial cues			Vocal cues	Cues to strength of feeling	Other (such as words used)
	Brows	Eyes	Mouth			
Angry						
Happy						
Sad						
Afraid						
Disgusted						
Interested /surprised						

Comments:

Discuss the exercise with reference to the discussion issues.

Discussion issues

1. What is the relative importance of verbal and non-verbal cues for the recognition of emotion?
2. Are there any particular cues that 'leak' true emotion?
3. Are there any particular emotions that (a) a nurse or (b) a patient might try to hide? (Use examples from your own experiences if possible.) If so, what are they, and what strategies are used to hide them?
4. What advantages or disadvantages are there in hiding real feelings as (a) a nurse, and (b) a patient?
5. Are some emotions more easily expressed than others? Why might this be?
6. What difficulties were there in doing this exercise?

Comments

consultant who we have known for years suddenly start biting her/his nails, we may be right in thinking that she/he is worried about something. Once again, it is the *change* from the person's usual way of behaving that is important.

We should notice, therefore, if patients start or stop doing something uncharacteristic, or if they behave in certain ways at particular times (for example, just before visiting) or in particular situations (for example, in the radiotherapy unit), as these changes in behaviour may reflect underlying concerns.

So, even if we accurately perceive or notice what is going on, we can only make sense of it if we understand the context in which it occurs. It is the failure to take the context into account that leads us to make mistakes in judging the inner feelings of others.

The context of emotion

Our understanding of the context is also important if we are to know when and where it is appropriate to express an emotion, and what the acceptable way of expressing that emotion will be. Why, for example, is it all right for a child to scream at the prospect of an injection, but not an adult; for a nurse to cry in the sluice room following a cardiac arrest, but not in front of the patients (or even other nurses); for a middle-aged man to weep for joy when he finds he does not have cancer, but not when he gets the dinner he ordered?

Display rules

There are rules that tell us when and how to express our feelings, depending on the culture and subcultures to which we belong. These rules are known as 'display rules' and are illustrated in Exercise 5.3.

They tell us when and how to display emotion. Different rules refer to the events that are 'allowed' to raise particular feelings, and the manner in which they should be expressed. There are, for example, differences between cultures in what emotion is experienced at death (joy/grief), and if the same emotion is produced — say grief — as to how it is expressed (quiet reserve/wailing/sobbing). We have to learn these rules as a part of being socialized into the culture to which we belong. Sometimes the learning is quite explicit (for example, when we tell children they are too big to be cross — or rather express anger — when their younger brother or sister takes the toy they were playing with), and sometimes the rules are picked up as we get more experienced (are we *told* that nurses should not cry?).

Emblematic behaviour

We also learn that sometimes facial expressions are used to communicate messages that have nothing to do with the expression of emotion, but rather that have a social meaning. When we pass the senior nursing officer in the corridor daily, and she/he raises her/his eyebrows as we pass we do not assume that she/he is constantly surprised to see us: rather, we know that raised eyebrows can be used as a form of greeting, instead of words (the message of raised eyebrows would be different if we saw someone 'doing it to us' from the

Exercise 5.3   Display rules and the expression of emotion

Instructions

Please think of a role from a nursing context (for example, nurse, patient, ward sister, doctor, relative, child, etc.) Write the title of the role in the space provided on the chart below. Please think about this particular role. Are there any circumstances wherein it would be *inappropriate* to express a particular emotion. Describe two situations for each emotion, and enter them on the chart. How do you know it would be inappropriate? Think of as many different ways we learn when and how to express emotions, and enter them on the chart.

Answer sheet

Role:

Feeling		*Inappropriate situation*	*Reasons for it being inappropriate*
Angry	1		
	2		
Sad	1		
	2		
Afraid	1		
	2		
Happy	1		
	2		
Interested/ surprised	1		
	2		
Disgusted	1		
	2		

Think about your answers in the light of the discussion issues.

Discussion issues

1. What is the importance of the context for the expression and recognition of emotions?
2. Does the recognition of an emotion differ from the interpretation of that emotion? If so, how?
3. How important is change in emotional expression?
4. Do people attempt to label or re-label their emotions according to the situation that they are in?

Comments

---

other side of the room at a party!) Used like this, facial expression is being used 'emblematically', and it is the context again that lets us know when a certain signal is being used to convey a particular feeling, or whether it is being used emblematically. If we confuse the two, we will make a mistake in interpreting what is going on.

Labelling emotional states

We use the context, too, to label an inner feeling we have as one emotion rather than another. It is the context then that makes us say we are nervous rather than thrilled when we are going to give our first injection, even though we would feel the same sensations as when we get the job we really wanted. Thus we label the emotion (and then express it differently) according to the context or situation we are in. In other words, our thought or cognitions about the situation we are in lead us to label the feelings we have.

We have looked, above, at the cues we use to recognize and express different emotional states, and at those cues that 'leak' information relating to inner feelings. We have considered the importance of the context in its relation to display rules, telling us when and how to express different emotions, and in labelling our own internal states. We will now go on to consider the nature of interpersonal attitudes and their role in interaction.

5.3 The recognition and expression of interpersonal attitudes

Feelings that we have towards other people are called interpersonal attitudes, and like emotions, we recognize them by what people do, rather than by what they say. In fact, in the course of our everyday lives we rarely tell someone exactly what we feel towards them, although we may leave them in little doubt.

We can think of our attitudes towards others as reflecting two central attitude dimensions, which are *friendly/warm* to *hostile/cold*, and *dominant/superior* to *submissive/inferior*. Thus, we relate to others in terms of liking or affiliation and status. Other common feelings we have are combinations of these two dimensions, and examples are:

boring	interesting	patronizing
pleasing	anxious	relaxing
tolerant	protective	defensive
despairing	frustrating	dependent

Although we use non-verbal information to judge another person's attitude towards us, the timing of a statement may also be a powerful way to communicate an attitude. Suffice it to say here, that if a patient were to say something unfriendly to us with a friendly expression on his/her face, and in a friendly tone of voice, then we would probably judge him/her as friendly. Interestingly, we are much better at knowing when other people like us than when they dislike us, and this may be because there is quite a lot of pressure not to show our negative feelings towards others.

No single non-verbal cue relates to a particular attitude. Rather, it is clusters of non-verbal behaviours that we respond to, with different clusters representing affiliative, hostile, dominant and submissive styles. In liking, for instance, the cues all bring us 'psychologically closer' to our partner, and are known as immediacy cues. A guide to the usual combinations of cues in the expression of liking and dominance is given in Table 5.2.

The context of interpersonal attitudes

We do not normally express what we feel, when we feel it, but rather decide how and what to communicate, depending on the situation. So, no matter how foolish we feel the hospital chaplain to be, we would probably not let him know that we felt superior; similarly, if we disliked colleagues on our ward,

Table 5.2　The expression of liking and dominance

Focus	Affiliative style	Dominant style
Face	Positive, e.g. interest, smiling	Relaxed, neutral or frowning
Gaze	Long and frequent looks; eye contact	Fewer but longer looks, breaks gaze last
Voice	Soft, low and resonant	Loud, deep tone
Distance	Fairly close (within three feet)	Either fairly close or fairly distant
Touch	Hand on arm	None
Position	About 45° angle	Directly in front
Posture	Open arms and either partially open or loosely crossed legs. Forward lean or moderate sideways lean	Reclining angle, relaxed limbs sprawled, shoulders squared, chest expanded
Orientation	Head and shoulders to each other	Either face to face or more than 45° away
Speech	Listener responses. Speaker disclosures of similarity. Few speech disturbances, good timing. Handing over conversations	Few reflections. Speaks at length. Quick responses and interruptions, asks questions and changes topics. Initiates and closes encounters, expresses different opinions

we might well let them know in various ways, but we would try to hide these feelings in front of patients.

As with emotions, there are cultural and subcultural differences in the expression of interpersonal attitudes. What we may think is a friendly approach, for example, may be interpreted as quite insulting, and vice versa. We will all have experienced the frustrations of being misunderstood by an older person, or indeed when we ourselves have misunderstood an older or younger person. A chance to explore the interpretation of interpersonal attitudes is given in Exercise 5.4.

Exercise 5.4   Interpretation of interpersonal attitudes

Instructions

Please collect a series of ten pictures of nurses at work, illustrating if possible, different attitudes towards other people. Look at each picture in turn and write down what you think the attitude being expressed is. Think about how you know what the attitude is, and write this in the chart. Repeat for each picture in turn. Discuss, if possible with a partner who has also completed the exercise, the discussion issues.

Answer sheet

Picture no.	What attitude was being expressed?	How do you know?
1		
2		
3		
4		
5		
6		
7		
8		
9		
10		

Discussion issues

1. Would there be different effects if the nurse in any of the target pictures was expressing that attitude to (a) a patient, (b) a more senior nurse?
2. Are there any cultural differences in the expression and recognition of interpersonal attitudes? If possible, give particular examples from your nursing experience.
3. What common misunderstandings have you encountered before? Give a particular example of an incident where you have been misunderstood or have misunderstood others. (Restrict your examples to those where the misunderstanding has been to do with the communication of interpersonal attitudes.)

Comments

Culture/subculture

It is important to realize some of the cultural differences in the communication of interpersonal attitudes, in order to avoid getting hold of the wrong end of the stick, and making mistakes. The Pakistani mother who appears diffident and unfriendly may be shy and unused to talking easily to strangers; the Rastafarian youth who appears indolent may just be adopting the style of behaviour common to his peer group. It can sometimes be very difficult for us to appreciate that another person's style of behaviour may not mean what we think it does, and we all have a tendency to jump to conclusions about the meaning of behaviour. This may well be because we are always on the lookout for some indication that other people like us and consider us to be their equal; this may make us over-sensitive to the smallest indication (often wrong) that they feel negatively towards us.

Roles

Roles often differ from each other in terms of status. We would not be particularly surprised or upset to find that the ward sister behaved as if she were more superior to her student nurses on the ward, as she has some legitimate superiority, in terms of seniority. If, however, she were to treat another sister or her nursing officer as inferior, this would be inappropriate. Similarly, if she met one of her student nurses on holiday, it would be inappropriate for her to act in a superior manner.

Thus, to make sense of interpersonal attitudes, we need to have an understanding of the culture/subculture to which people belong, the role they occupy and the situation they are in, as well as being able to perceive and interpret different clusters of non-verbal behaviours.

Once we have understood the emotion or interpersonal attitude being expressed, we must be able to communicate that understanding, if we are to develop a rapport with our partner, and it is the communication of understanding that we will go on to consider.

5.4 The communication of understanding

The most common way we communicate understanding is by listening to what our partner is telling us. When we listen we do not just sit passively while our partner talks, we actively let him/her know that she/he is being attended to, heard and understood.

Listening

We use different listening skills on different occasions and for different purposes, and our behaviour varies along a dimension of activity. Sometimes, it is enough for us to sit quietly still, alert, looking in the general direction of our partner, and engaging in direct eye contact. If, however, we did this in casualty when a distraught mother was giving us a garbled account of her child's accident we would neither get the information we need, nor calm the mother. In nursing, a lot of conversations take place whilst other tasks are being carried out, and at these times we would need to engage in more active and pronounced listening. So, in listening to a patient complain about the physiotherapy programme whilst we are concentrating on removing some stitches, we might use small vocalizations (mmm, uh huh, oh, I see, etc.) and pronounced gestures such as head nods. This is known as minimal listening, and we must be careful that we do not slip into minimum attention, go into 'automatic pilot', and cease really to respond to our patient.

When we listen to somebody who is obviously emotional, we need to be more active still, and use the skill of reflecting. Basically, reflecting is the ability to let our partner know that we really have heard both the factual and emotional content of what they have said, or communicated non-verbally. We have to be careful when we reflect, not merely to repeat what the person had said word for word, as to talk to a 'parrot' is at best irritating and at worst insulting and unpleasant. True reflections are difficult to do well, and it is a good idea to practise paraphrasing what people say, and finding a few words that sum up quite complicated feelings. Listening skills are explored in Exercise 5.5.

Exercise 5.5   Listening

Instructions

With a partner, or with two other people, allocate the roles, A, B and O (A — speaker; B — listener; O — observer).

1. A — Briefly describe what you did last Saturday afternoon.
   B — Communicate to A that you have heard what she/he said, and that you understand it.
   O — Note down those signals B used to show A that she/he really was listening. How did she/he communicate (a) attention, (b) understanding?
   Discuss any issues raised as a result of doing this task.
   A and O give B any advice you can, about how she/he could have been a 'better' listener.
2. Swop roles.
   A — Briefly describe the last time you felt really happy about something.
   B — Communicate to A that you have heard what she/he said, and that you understand it.
   O — Note down those signals B used to show A that she/he really was listening. How did she/he communicate (a) attention, (b) understanding the content, and (c) understanding the feeling?
   Discuss any issues raised as a result of doing this task.
   A and O give B any advice you can about how she/he could have been a 'better' listener.
3. Swop roles.
   A — Briefly describe a situation where another person has made you irritated or angry. What did she/he do, and what did you do as a result?
   B — Communicate to A that you have heard what she/he said, that you understand it, and that you sympathize with the way she/he handled the situation.
   O — Note down those signals that B used to show A that she/he really was listening. How did she/he communicate (a) attention, (b) understanding the content, (c) understanding the feeling, and (d) appreciation of the solution.
   Discuss any issues raised as a result of doing this task.
   A and O give B any advice you can about how she/he could have been a 'better' listener.
4. Discuss with each other the fundamental aspects of effective listening with reference to the discussion issues.

Discussion issues

1. Is it possible to be over-attentive? If so, what effect does this have?
2. Are there any situations where the level of listening is unimportant?
3. What feelings does not being listened to arouse?
4. What is the importance of feedback in conversations?
5. Were there any difficulties in accurately expressing and recognizing feelings?

Comments

In some situations, particularly if someone is finding it difficult to tell us something, we may need to ask questions as part of our listening technique. Questions are part of a listening skill when they are used to encourage our partners to continue or to elaborate on what they were saying. For example, the mother of a twelve-year-old tonsillectomy patient may be ashamed to tell us of his nocturnal enuresis, but if it is recognized that she wants to tell us something, and is encouraged to do so, we may all save the boy himself from considerable embarrassment and discomfort.

At times, we may want to offer a personal commentary on what people say, again to encourage them to speak or to think of things connected to what they are saying that they might otherwise not have thought of. It can be very reassuring and comforting for distressed patients to know our own feelings or beliefs about what they are saying, or for colleagues to know that we have experienced feelings similar to those that they are expressing. As long as the commentary is used to make it easier for our partner to talk further, it is still a listening skill.

Thus we can see that the more active the listening, the more it requires us to speak! Listening skills are developed in Section 8.2.

Empathy

If we are to be really effective listeners, we must develop the ability to 'take the role of the other', or see things from the other person's shoes. If we are able to do this, we can empathize with that person. It is easy to confuse empathy with sympathy, and indeed, we use many of the same techniques in the communication of both empathy and sympathy. Many of the non-verbal behaviours we use to reassure patients, such as close proximity, prolonged eye contact, touch, calm soothing voice, etc. are all part of empathy, but often, in addition, we will say something as well. We have mentioned reflections above, and these can be used to communicate empathy; however, we can communicate 'advanced empathy' by attempting to draw threads between different conversations, or point to themes that emerge over several occasions, and suggest connections that our partners may not have thought of for themselves. This technique is similar to some of those used in social problem solving (see Sections 7.1 and 8.2), but when we use it to convey empathy, we are concerned with the emotional content of the conversation. Advanced empathy is particularly important when we are involved with another person over some time in what may be seen as a counselling relationship.

Touch

Touch is a signal that is of great significance for us in nursing, both because we use it a lot in just carrying out many nursing tasks, and because if we use it judicially in times of emotional distress, it can be a powerful empathic tool. We are often unaware of how and when we touch people, and Exercise 5.6 provides the opportunity to examine these issues.

We are often required, for both active listening and empathy, to reveal things about ourselves, that is, to engage in self-disclosure, and indeed, when and how much to disclose is a very big problem for us as nurses, and when we think about it the issue becomes one of how and if we should keep our role boundaries.

5.5 Self-disclosure

Self-disclosure refers to the verbal aspects of self-presentation, and particularly to information about ourselves that others could not share if we did not reveal it. Thus self-disclosure differs from self-description, which refers to the information that other people can easily get about us (for example, I am a staff nurse, I am 30 years old, and so on). We can disclose factual information (I have been in hospital), emotions (I am afraid of anaesthetics), general feelings (I like people), or specific feelings (I like Sister Evans). Disclosures can be used as part of empathy, and can be varied according to whether they are *genuine* or *apparent*. Genuine disclosures are those of a personal nature that we may find embarrassing to reveal, so when we do, it is an indication that we trust the recipient of the information, and since trust is generally thought to be rewarding, this is likely to lead to greater

Exercise 5.6 Touch

Instructions

Please look at the descriptions on each of the front-back pairs of figures below. Shade in those areas that it would be appropriate for you, as a nurse, to touch that person. Use darker shading for more frequent touching.

Answer sheet

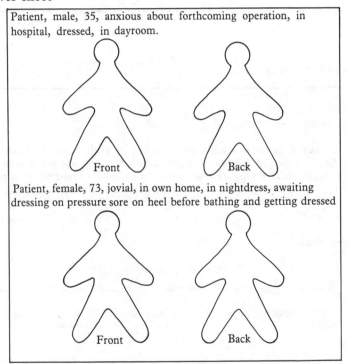

Patient, male, 35, anxious about forthcoming operation, in hospital, dressed, in dayroom.

Front   Back

Patient, female, 73, jovial, in own home, in nightdress, awaiting dressing on pressure sore on heel before bathing and getting dressed

Front   Back

Consider the results of shading in the light of the discussion issues.

Discussion issues

1. Would your shading have been different if the target figures had been fifteen years younger/from a different culture/well known to you?
2. Are there any types of people or particular illnesses that people have that make it difficult for you to touch them? Why do you think this is?

3. Is it easier/more difficult to touch a patient if other nursing staff are around? Why is this?
4. Can you think of any examples where patients have touched you, as a nurse, either appropriately or inappropriately?

Comments

Exercise 5.7   Self-disclosure

Instructions

Please give two examples of self-disclosures to fit each of the categories in the chart below. Each category differs in terms of its intimacy and whether it is about a positive/negative/neutral topic. (Please note that these are *dimensions* where increasing intimacy is represented: they are not completely separate categories.)

Answer sheet

Degree of intimacy

Non-intimate........................moderately intimate...............intimate...........................

Positive	Kind of group activity I enjoy 1. 2.	The kind of people I find it easy to talk to 1. 2.	My good reputation with others 1. 2.
Neutral	Whether or not I laugh at dirty jokes 1. 2.	Which I value more friendship or money 1. 2.	Things I don't like to talk about with others 1. 2.
Negative	My aversion to crowds 1. 2.	Things that annoy me about others 1. 2.	Things that would cause me to break up a friendship 1. 2.

Consider your answers in the light of the discussion issues.

Discussion issues

1. Are there cultural differences in the use of self-disclosures? Give examples if possible.
2. When does self-disclosure become boasting?
3. Is reciprocity of self-disclosure necessary? What problems might this raise for nurses?
4. Does being a nurse encourage or discourage specific self-disclosures? Give specific examples.
5. What are the 'dangers' of self-disclosing as a nurse?
6. Are there any facets of 'self' that it is acceptable for nurses to ask of patients, but not to consider revealing themselves?
7. What are the advantages of self-disclosure?
8. What is the relevance of the context for self-disclosure?

Comments

_____

intimacy. We use apparent disclosures in situations where the sharing of information (rather than feeling) is expected. Apparent disclosures are not particularly embarrassing, and result in the experience of a pleasant encounter, rather than the development of trust. Since we experience both trust and reciprocity (sharing) as rewarding, both types of disclosures help the development of rapport, but this will rarely happen if disclosures are one-sided. Exercise 5.7 seeks to clarify the different types of self-disclosure.

We may feel, though, that the demands and expectations relating to the role of nurse make it inappropriate for us to use many genuine disclosures in our work. We may find, for example, that patients readily talk about their sex problems (genuine disclosure) to us as nurses, but we feel that it would be inappropriate to share with them our own sexual problems — or would it?

The context of self-disclosure

The use of self-disclosure does not always lead to the development of a rapport. If it is not the right time or place to divulge certain information, we may find that the people we are talking to become uncomfortable and end up disliking us. Patients who talk at meal-time, for example about the pain they feel in passing urine, are likely to cause embarrassment and to be disliked. When we are considering the value of particular self-disclosures, we also need to know something about the norms or rules that underlie the acceptability of self-disclosure in different situations.

Rules

There are also rules relating to whether we should reveal positive or negative information about ourselves, even of an impersonal nature (apparent disclosure). We are more likely to develop a rapport with new colleagues if they tell us about the kind of holiday they enjoy, rather than their aversion to people snoring, when we first meet them! Generally, we will embarrass people if we reveal either intimate or negative information about ourselves early in the relationship, and this will hinder the development of rapport.

There is an age-old belief that nurses should take care to 'protect' themselves and not get too involved with patients, and remain detached. By not using self-disclosures, we will be better at keeping our distance, but this may be at the expense of not allowing ourselves to develop rapport with patients. This may, in turn, mean that we are not as helpful to patients as we could be. Rather than ensuring we keep this distance, we might find that we (and patients) experience less distress and more satisfaction if we allow ourselves the freedom to choose when and where to use self-disclosures. Our task will then be one of judging the appropriateness of a disclosure and of striking a balance between the positive effects of conveying empathy and developing rapport, and the negative effects of over-involvement.

Of course, self-disclosures are threatening, as there is always the possibility that our 'real' selves will not be liked; and this is especially true of genuine disclosures. We should bear this in mind when patients or colleagues have summoned up the courage to tell us something they think is personally important, and we feel the urge to treat it lightly.

5.6 Summary

This chapter has been concerned with the skills that are needed to establish and maintain rapport in interaction, that is with facilitation skills. Specifically, the following issues were raised:

Facilitation skills are used to develop and maintain rapport.

If rapport is to develop, interactions must be rewarding.

The accurate recognition and expression of emotions and interpersonal attitudes are central to the establishment of rapport, and to ensuring that interaction will be rewarding.

There is often a discrepancy between the recognition and interpretation of emotions and interpersonal attitudes.

The change from a person's usual way of behaving is the key to understanding the meaning of her/his behaviour.

Emotions and interpersonal attitudes can only be fully understood if the social context is taken into account.

The social context determines the display rules of emotional expression, and gives information regarding the norms that dictate how and when to reveal interpersonal attitudes and to use self-disclosure.

Listening is one of the most important facilitation skills.

Effective listening varies from less active to more active, that is from giving attention to using minimal vocalisations to reflecting the verbal and emotional content of the message to asking questions to giving a personal commentary.

The more active the listening, the more likely that empathy is conveyed.

Empathy includes the willingness to self-disclose.

Self-disclosures may be of information or feeling; they may be genuine or apparent; and may be positive or negative.

The social context (including roles and relationships) determines the appropriateness of a disclosure.

Appropriate disclosures are rewarding and strengthen relationships. Inappropriate disclosures are embarrassing and weaken relationships.

Further reading

Argyle, M. (1982) *The Psychology of Interpersonal Behaviour* (4th edn), Penguin, Harmondsworth

Egan, G. (1981) *The Skilled Helper* (2nd edn), Brooks Cole, New York

French, P. (1983) *Social Skills for Nursing Practice*, Croom Helm, London

Gahagan, J. (1984) *Social Interaction and Its Management*, Methuen, London

Jourard, S. (1971) *Self-Disclosure: an experimental analysis of the transparent self*, Wiley, New York

Smith, V.M. and Bass, T.A. (1982) *Communication for the Health Care Team*, Harper and Row, London

Tschudin, V. (1982) *Counselling Skills for Nurses*, Baillière Tindall, London

CHAPTER 6

CONTROL AND ASSERTION

Chapter 5 was concerned with the concept of rewardingness in interactions, underlying facilitation skills. In Figure I we can see that this is only one set of skills that can be mustered in response to our goals for a particular interaction. The other skills are those associated with assertion and control. In this chapter we will examine the place of control in social interaction generally, and go on to consider, specifically:

(a) the use of questions in interpersonal control
(b) the giving of information and explanation, and
(c) assertiveness.

6.1 Control and social interaction

Interpersonal relationships may be seen as systems of mutual influence. In even the most casual interactions, 'speakers' control 'listeners' by talking, so that they have to listen, and vice versa. Influence may be uneven in more formal situations, due to the different roles that people have. Sometimes the circumstances may require that overt — even physical — control is exercised. The notion of control in the context of interpersonal skills, therefore, ranges from subtle influence with little conscious intent to overt and deliberate direction and regulation of others. The focus of the influence may be on other people's behaviour, their thoughts or their feelings. In other words, our social behaviour (verbal and non-verbal) will affect how others consequently think or feel.

Control is wielded by everyone in a social situation to some degree. Nurses control patients by asking them questions, issuing them with instructions, giving them explanations or information, reassuring them or even by just passing the time of day with them. Patients control nurses, for example, by asking *them* questions, withholding or volunteering information, complimenting or criticizing them, or refusing to take medication. Nurses also control colleagues in a variety of ways and for a variety of reasons.

We have seen how conversations can be regulated through the use of listening skills (Exercises 3.3, 5.5), particularly those depending on non-verbal strategies. Skilled use of verbal strategies, as part of more complex listening skills also serve to regulate conversation. Questioning, probing, clarification and elaboration skills can all be used to elicit conversation and to encourage a speaker to explore a range of experiences, and Exercise 6.1 provides a chance to practise these skills.

In Exercise 6.1 a variety of different techniques will have been used to help the 'speaker' recall his/her experience. Many of these will have used different sorts of questions, and we propose now to examine questioning as a means of control more closely.

Questions and interpersonal control

We have seen (Section 4.3) that questions may be used to open conversations and initiate social interaction. They may also be used to elicit personal and medical information, to ascertain attitudes, opinions and feelings, to show interest in a topic or another person, to identify needs, to assess a person's knowledge or understanding, to help conversations go smoothly, to encourage exploration of experiences and to direct action. A summary of the social functions of questioning is given in Table 6.1.

These functions are not mutually exclusive and a particular question may serve more than one of them. Take, for example, a nurse asking a patient, 'How comfortable are you?' This may be a conversation opening of various sorts, an attempt to obtain information, part of patient assessment or a means of identifying the patient's needs. We can only know the function of a question by examining it in the interaction context. Thus the function of 'How comfortable are you?' will depend on whether it comes at the beginning of the conversation and if not, what went before, and so on.

Exercise 6.1   Speech elicitation

Instructions

In pairs label yourselves A and B. Person A go out of the room and walk about for 3–4 minutes. Person B turn to page 334 and read the instructions to B there (this exercise will not be very useful if both A and B read the instructions before undertaking the task.) When A returns tell B about your experience out of the room. When you have discussed this experience for as long as possible consider the discussion issues. B should tell A what her/his instructions had been.

Discussion issues

1. How easy was this exercise for A and B? Why?
2. What non-verbal strategies did B use?
3. What verbal strategies did B use?
4. Which strategies were the most helpful for A?
5. Would different strategies be of more use in different situations? Which and why?
6. Are there any examples from your nursing experience where similar strategies for eliciting speech from other people might be used?

Comments

Table 6.1 Functions of questions

1. To initiate interaction

Casual, informal openings	N.	Hello, you're new aren't you?
	P.	Have you got a minute, please?
To arouse interest/motivation	N.	Who do you think is coming to see you this afternoon?
	P.	Nurse — should the blood be coming up the tube like this?
To show interest and concern	N.	Are you all right in there?
	P.	What are you so happy about?
To orientate a task group	N.	Is everyone clear what we are doing this afternoon?

2. To obtain information

Facts	N.	Have you had any illness in childhood?
	N.	Do you have someone to bring in your things for you?
	P.	When will the doctors be round?
	P.	What is that drip for?
Attitudes/feelings/opinions	N.	How do you feel about going home so soon?
	N.	What do you think about the physiotherapy sessions?
	P.	Would you let your child have the whooping cough jab?
	P.	What do you think about epidurals?

3. To guide conversation

Change the subject	N.	I see, but when did you first feel uncomfortable?
	P.	I understand that lunch is at 12, but when am I going to scan?
Encourage thought about the future	N.	How do you think your husband will cope when you go home?
	P.	Who will do it for me when you are off next week?

Assessment	N.	How has your family taken the news?
	P.	Have you changed one of these dressings before?
Clarification	N.	What is it you're worried about?
	P.	Do you want me to roll my sleeve right up?
Clarification of jargon	N.	When you said you were *confused*, what did you mean?
	P.	You said I had an oedematous knee: what did you mean?
Manipulation	N.	I think we should leave this just now don't you?
	P.	You're not up to dealing with people like me are you?

4. To identify problems and needs

Precision	N.	When, exactly, did these anxious feelings start?
	P.	How long will I have to wait for the results?
Judge extent of existing knowledge	N.	Why do you (think) you take these particular drugs?
	P.	Did the receptionist tell you why I'm here?
Confront emotion	N.	You sound very angry: would you like to tell me why?
	P.	You look fed up: would you rather talk some other time?
Check understanding	N.	So, after what I've just told you, will you just run over the procedure for giving yourself the injection?
	P.	When will I be able to see you again, after my holiday?
Memory	N.	Do you remember how to use the machine?
	P.	What did I ask you?

5. To expand previous points
   (probing)

Clarification	N. How exactly does you asthma affect you at work?
Relevance to other issues	N. Does your breathing get worse in smoky rooms?
	N. How crucial do you think anxiety is in sparking off an attack?
Extension	N. Is there anything else you can tell me about when your asthma occurs?
Accuracy	N. Did you say your breathing was worse at night?
Consensus	N. You disagree about whether her wheezing is better when it's warm: can you come to some agreement about this?

6. To guide action

Requests	N. Can I take some blood from you now?
	P. Please may I make another appointment?
Commands	N. Would you like to go back to your bed now, please?
	N. Please will you just roll over so I can do the other side?
	P. Would you be so good as to hold the door open?

We have seen (Section 3.2) that some conversation strategies are part of social routines and ritual, and do not, in themselves, mean what they appear to. Questions are frequently subject to this ambiguity. Thus, a command issued in the form of a question, such as, 'Would you like to take these pills now, please?' appears to offer choice, when none was intended. Similarly a routine question such as 'Everything all right, here?' may invite a detailed reply, when it was intended as a social pleasantry. Exercise 6.2 considers different types of questions.

Questions are used for different purposes in different situations, and not all the functions will always be relevant. The reasons for using questions at home or in informal social settings will be different from at work. The way in which a question is asked in part determines how well it serves the function that was intended. There are different types of questions that lead to different types of replies, and that are more or less useful. Much of the research into the verbal behaviour of nurses indicates that nurses tend to use inappropriate styles of questioning that result in failures of communication from both their own and the patients' point of view. Patients are not given the opportunity to explore their feelings, while nurses fail to detect underlying needs and frequently miss the opportunity to gather vital information.

Questions can be *open* or *closed*, and it is the situation, coupled with the goals of the questions that determine which style is most appropriate.

Closed questions are ones that limit the possibilities of reply. They are used in the collection of facts and to discover preferences between given alternatives: frequently they invite yes/no answers, and thus do not encourage much talk. The questioner requires prior knowledge about the topic of conversation, in order to decide on the most useful question(s) to ask. Because of this, though, valuable information may be lost if she/he has limited knowledge or considers some topics to be unimportant or insignificant. Many situations require the use of closed questions, for example, 'What drugs are you taking?'; 'Who is your G.P.?'; 'Would you like the light off now?'; 'Is yours the blue or the red towel?'; 'Has the pain gone?'

Open questions, on the other hand, allow the respondent the freedom to reply in any way she/he wishes. They encourage talk as yes/no answers are difficult to make. Because the onus is on the respondent to provide detail, little prior knowledge of the topic is required of the questioner. This means though, that if the respondent considers information to be unimportant or insignificant, it may well be lost. As the content of the reply is unpredictable, the questioner needs considerable skill in taking up cues in order to pursue the conversation meaningfully, and to avoid becoming sidetracked. Open

Exercise 6.2   Functions of questions

Instructions

Please write down a question you have asked or have been asked during the past week either at home or at work. With reference to Table 6.1 try to identify the functions that question served and write them in the table below. If you cannot find an appropriate function in Table 6.1 describe the function of the question as best you can.

Answer sheet

Question 1   Function

Question 2   Function

Question 3   Function

Question 4   Function

Question 5   Function

Question 6   Function

Question 7   Function

Question 8   Function

Question 9   Function

Question 10   Function

With a partner who has also completed the exercise, if possible, consider the discussion issues.

Discussion issues

1. Were any different functions served by questions from the two contexts? Why?
2. Was it difficult to find examples of any of the functions? Why?
3. Did any functions emerge that were not included in the original list? Add to Table 6.1.

Comments

questions are particularly valuable in eliciting attitudes, values, opinions and feelings, and as such may be threatening to either party (which may be one reason why nurses seem reluctant to use them to their full extent). Some examples of open questions would be, 'How did you twist your ankle?'; 'How do you feel about the operation now?'; 'How have your children been?'; 'What do you think about that?'

Both closed and open questions can be useful in nurse–patient interaction. There is, as we have said, a tendency to use closed questions when open ones would have been more appropriate. Indeed, closed questions undoubtedly give the *questioner* control over both the conversation and his/her emotional involvement. It is useful to be able to distinguish clearly between closed and open questions and to practise both kinds, so that we can use them to their best effect, and Exercise 6.3 offers the chance to do this.

There are other types of questions that are in common use but that have little positive value. They control and determine the course of the interaction and leave the respondents with perceptions and feelings about the questioner that are generally unintended. Sometimes, though, the effects they have *are* intended, in which case they serve a manipulative function. Leading questions are those whose wording suggests the answer that is expected. Most leading questions invite the respondent to agree with a statement of fact or value contained within the question. For example:

There's no need to be afraid of injections, is there?
You're feeling better today, then?'
Most of our men in here don't have anything for pain: do you need something?
This is a nice friendly ward, isn't it?

Leading questions can be more subtle, encouraging the acceptance of certain premises and thereby limiting the possibilities of reply. Consider variations of the above:

How scared of injections are you?
How much better do you feel?
How do you cope with your pain?
Do you find everyone friendly?

In these examples, the questions are loaded in a particular direction and thus encourage only certain replies. Similar bias is produced by questions that lead a respondent to reply as she/he thinks she/he should, with reference to prestigious or normative values, at the expense of honesty. Questions such as, 'How often do you wash your hair at home?', 'Does she have vegetables every day?', 'What time does she go to bed?' may produce a very misleading picture of a child's home routine. The problem with questions like these is that the respondent assumes the norm, and thus may bias her/his reply in unpredictable ways.

Questions that may leave the respondent confused, and elicit misinformative replies are those that in effect ask several things at once. Sometimes they may be double-barrelled (for example, 'Are you in pain or nauseated?') or multi-faceted (for example, 'Do you shiver or perspire or get cramp or vomit or fall asleep?'). The respondent may want to reply to some/all/none of the alternatives.

The final type of question that is often ambiguous and thereby confusing, is the rhetorical question. Rhetorical questions are really statements and do not require an answer. They are used in conversation as opening and closing gambits, and sometimes defensively in the course of the conversation, with the questioner subsequently providing the answer. The trouble is, sometimes people reply to them! 'Lovely day, isn't it?' 'What shall we do with you — Send you to X-ray?' are examples of rhetorical questions.

The different types of questions are summarized in Table 6.2.

We have seen, then, that questions are not simply requests for information. They serve many different functions, and the skilled choice of style of questioning can ensure that nurses get all they can from interviews with patients, relatives and colleagues. The context or situation will determine what it is that nurses hope to get out of their conversations, and their goals should determine their choice of questioning style.

Just as nurses can control interactions through the skilled use of questions, so too can patients. Calls for explanation, information and (sometimes) reassurance are often made, and nurses have to respond to them.

Exercise 6.3   Open and closed questions

Instructions

Complete Exercise 6.2. Using the questions that were collected in Exercise 6.2, please re-write each of the questions in *open* and *closed* styles. Indicate the likely effects of each style on interaction.

Answer sheet

Question 1   Effect on interaction
Open
Closed

Question 2   Effect on interaction
Open
Closed

Question 3   Effect on interaction
Open
Closed

Question 4   Effect on interaction
Open
Closed

Question 5   Effect on interaction
Open
Closed

Question 6   Effect on interaction
Open
Closed

Question 7   Effect on interaction
Open
Closed

Question 8   Effect on interaction
Open
Closed

Instructions

In order to think more about the differences between styles of questions it is useful to distinguish between those that focus on feeling and facts and that differ in how specific they are. The chart below represents three ways that questions can differ from each other:

Open/Closed; Fact/Feeling; General/Specific.

Please give two examples of each of the eight types of questions. Write your examples in the appropriate boxes. Try to ensure that the examples are ones that may be heard in nursing settings.

Answer sheet

	Open		*Closed*	
	Facts	*Feelings*	*Facts*	*Feelings*
General				
1.	What are you interested in?	How do you feel now?	Have you been in hospital before?	Are you comfortable?
2.				
3.				
Specific				
1.	What did you daughter say when you told her?	You seem angry, would you like to tell me about it?	Have you been on this ward before?	Do you feel angry now?
2.				
3.				

With a partner who has also completed the exercise, if possible, consider the discussion issues.

Discussion issues

1. Are some types of questions more common in nursing settings than others? Why might this be?
2. Was it difficult to find examples of any particular type of question?
3. Are there some situations where closed questions are more appropriate than open questions or vice versa?
4. Why do nurses tend to avoid using open questions?
5. What consequences do open questions have for (a) the questioner and (b) the respondent?
6. What other interpersonal skills are required if (a) open and (b) closed questions are to be used effectively?

Comments

Information and explanation

Nurses often respond to requests for information with attempts to reassure the patients. Comments such as 'It won't hurt,' 'You'll be all right don't worry' are rife, in the (false) belief that such consolation will help patients cope, and presumably aid recovery: they rarely do. In offering this false reassurance nurses stand in danger of dismissing patients' distress as part of normal processes rather than as genuine expressions of concerns. Take, for example, platitudes such as 'I'm sure it's uncomfortable, it always is at this stage' or 'Everyone finds it difficult to sleep when they first come in — you'll get over it.' It is, sometimes, appropriate to give reassurance. However, it will only be effective if nurses first establish what the patient is concerned about and why. If reassurance is used by the nurses as a means of avoiding underlying concerns, it will do little to help the patient.

More commonly, a request that at first appears to be for reassurance is really one for explanation or information. Patients often ask for information about medical/hospital activities and procedure, the nature of their disease, treatment and prognosis, as well as the reasons for their current feelings. The

Table 6.2   Types of questions or styles of questioning

Helpful styles
   Used appropriately, fulfil many social functions

Closed questions
Limit the possibilities of reply
Useful in eliciting facts; when selection between alternatives is required; when yes/no
   answers are appropriate
Questioner needs prior knowledge
Discourages talk
Non-threatening (usually)

Open questions
Provide the freedom to answer in any way
Useful in eliciting attitudes, values, feelings, opinions
Little prior knowledge required
Encourages talk
May be threatening

Unhelpful styles
   Create ambiguity and confusion

Leading questions
Wording suggests answer
Statement and/or value contained in question
Encourages the acceptance of premises in subtle ways
May invite respondent to bias answer to reflect (assumed) normative values
Misleading replies may be given as a result question rather than respondents' intent

Double-barrelled/multifaceted questions
Two or more questions asked as one
Respondent may want to reply to all/some/none of the alternatives

Rhetorical questions
Statements posed as questions: no answer generally required
Questioner may go on to provide the answer
Respondent may (mistakenly) provide an answer

---

need to give information stems also from nurses. Nurses may want to explain procedures and possible outcomes in order to prepare patients, say, for tests or surgery etc.; they may want to gain patients' cooperation with nursing tasks or to teach them how to undertake the tasks themselves, or they may be responsible for notifying patients of test results and their implications. It can be seen, then, that the *need* for information may stem from patients or nurses or both, and it is necessary to be clear about the origin of the need in order to plan and present the information to its best effect.

Figure 6.1 outlines the *process* of giving effective information. We often fall into the trap of giving explanations prematurely, and of providing too much information at once. It is necessary, therefore to *check* the extent of the recipient's knowledge in order to plan what to say and how. At the *planning* stage, several questions need to be asked. First, will the explanation be written, spoken, recorded or 'live'? Of course some situations require immediate verbal response to a request, in which case this choice may not exist: others, though, permit planning in advance. Second, what are the essential points to be covered and in what order? If the order of importance of points is not carefully considered, then problems of misunderstanding may arise as issues relating to diagnosis, treatment, side effects and prognosis become intermingled. Third, what illustrations or examples will be used to make the explanation more clear and/or memorable? Fourth, what constraints (such as hospital regulations, sister's instructions, doctors' rules, etc.) dictate what can and cannot be said?

Whether the information is prepared in advance or is offered spontaneously, there are several things to be borne in mind in *presenting* it.

Figure 6.2 shows the steps involved in effective information giving. The first relevant point is chosen and related as precisely and accurately as possible in a language style (see Section 3.2) that is appropriate to the particular recipient. After that, elaboration in the form of anecdote, analogy, or illustration may be given, again in a form that is familiar and in an appropriate style. In order to monitor the appropriate speed and amount of information, continual checks on understanding and/or acceptance should be made. This can be done by paying careful attention to non-verbal cues, and asking questions such as 'Is there any part of what I said that you'd like me to go over?'; 'Would you repeat what I've said so far?'; 'How does what I've told you make you feel?' As a result of the checking process it may be appropriate to reiterate previous points, stop the explanation for the time being or clarify again the point that was being made. Only after further checking has revealed that the point is understood should the explanation proceed. (Clearly, this

Figure 6.1   The process of giving information: nurse (N.) to patient (P.)

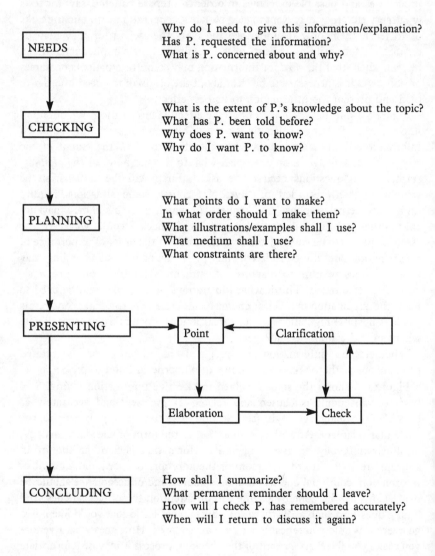

NEEDS
> Why do I need to give this information/explanation?
> Has P. requested the information?
> What is P. concerned about and why?

CHECKING
> What is the extent of P.'s knowledge about the topic?
> What has P. been told before?
> Why does P. want to know?
> Why do I want P. to know?

PLANNING
> What points do I want to make?
> In what order should I make them?
> What illustrations/examples shall I use?
> What medium shall I use?
> What constraints are there?

PRESENTING → Point ← Clarification
Point → Elaboration → Check
Clarification → Check → (back to Clarification)

CONCLUDING
> How shall I summarize?
> What permanent reminder should I leave?
> How will I check P. has remembered accurately?
> When will I return to discuss it again?

Figure 6.2 Presentation of information

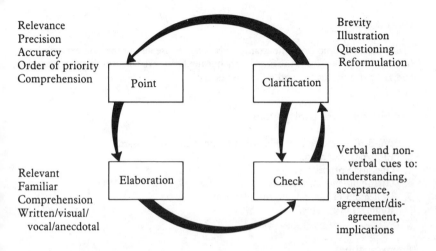

checking or clarification process cannot be done in quite the same way when the information is in written form. However, some attempt should still be made to answer any queries about, or clarify, written explanations.)

The final stage of the process is that of *concluding*. This may involve summarizing what has been said; further checking for understanding; establishing the need, and, if relevant, the time and place for a follow-up session; and leaving a permanent reminder of the major points that had been made. The process of giving information can be practised in Exercise 6.4.

During Exercise 6.4 it is likely that some of the common faults that nurses make in giving information will have emerged. We will, now, briefly summarize these faults.

Lack of structure at the planning and presenting stages may lead to poor use of time and involve the nurse in *needless repetition*. To a certain extent, this can be avoided by outlining the proposed explanation and interspersing it with constant checks for understanding. The inadvertent *use of technical language* or jargon may contribute to misunderstanding or ambiguity. Sometimes, unfortunately, nurses use jargon deliberately, as a defensive strategy that prevents patients questioning them further and more deeply about emotionally laden topics. Exercise 6.5 highlights some of the problems of using jargon and technical language when giving information.

Exercise 6.4   Giving information

Instructions

Please select a topic from the examples below. Devise an appropriate explanation to be given to a patient. Use the framework outlined below to construct your explanation, and refer to Figures 6.1 and 6.2 as necessary.

Sample topics for explanations

1. Ward routine to a new admission on an orthopaedic ward.
2. Electrocardiograph.
3. Operative procedure.
4. Giving an enema.
5. Collection of mid-stream sample of urine.
6. Removal of sutures.

Answer sheet

Topic of information

1. *Needs*   (Identify up to 3 needs to provide this information)

    (a)
    (b)
    (c)

2. *Checking*   (List 3 questions you might want to ask of the person, initially)

    (a)
    (b)
    (c)

3. *Planning*   (List the major points you want to make, and note some appropriate illustrations)

Points	Illustrations

    (a)
    (b)
    (c)
    (d)
    (e)

What medium will you use? (written/pictorial/spoken etc.)
What constraints might there be?

(a)
(b)
(c)

4. *Presenting*   (Construct your explanation and prepare to present it in the chosen medium)

(a)
(b)
(c)

5. *Concluding*   (List 3 actions you will take in conclusion)

(a)
(b)
(c)

6. *Comments*

With a partner who has also completed the exercise, if possible, discuss your explanation with reference to the discussion issues.

Discussion issues

1. How could this information be improved?
2. Would the information be different if the recipient was a relative rather than the patient? Why?
3. How could the information be modified for older/younger patients?
4. What would be the most appropriate form of checking?
5. Are you any the wiser? Why/why not?

Comments

Exercise 6.5   Jargon and technical language

Instructions

Please re-write the following explanations in a style that is free from jargon and technical language.

Answer sheet

1. *First-year student nurse to elderly patient:* I am going to administer an enema in order to evacuate your rectum and lower bowel of impacted faeces. Try to retain the enema for as long as possible. To facilitate this we'll elevate the end of your bed.
    Re-write:

2. *Ward sister to footballer prior to meniscectomy:* You'll need to fast for 6 hours prior to surgery, because the contents of your stomach may be vomited or regurgitated during some period of the anaesthesia, and inadvertently inhaled in the absence of your cough reflex.
    Re-write:

3. *Staff nurse to teenage mother of baby with gastro-enteritis:* We're going to take precautions to control the spread of cross-infection. This will include isolation and special disposal of all contaminated equipment.
    Re-write:

   With a partner who has also completed the exercise, if possible, consider the discussion issues.

Discussion issues

1. Would the re-write be different if the contexts of the explanations were different? How?
2. To what extent was the re-write specifically tailored to the roles of the people involved?
3. How would the explanations be changed if they were to be given to children?

Comments

Understanding is also inhibited if an *inappropriate style of speech* is adopted. If nurses speak in an unfamiliar restricted code, the patient may not attend to, or remember, what has been said. Again, checking for understanding should indicate when the style is wrong or further clarifiction is necessary. This may be particularly important when talking to patients from other regions/cultures about medical matters where frequent use of euphemism is made. It is just as unhelpful to give *poor illustrations* with reference to unfamiliar examples or analogies; what is obvious to one person may be quite obscure to another, and nurses can then find themselves side-tracked into explaining the illustration!

If insufficient attention is paid to how explanations are given, the information may well be *inaccurate*. Inaccuracy occurs unintentionally (as, for example, when nurses are unaware of their insufficient knowledge or when they unwittingly include personal opinion/values, as if they were facts), or deliberately, in the name of patients' interest. When the truth is distorted and shrouded in medical terminology, it is often when the information is negative and likely to be traumatic. When nurses use 'ulcer' or 'cyst' when they mean cancer, they have lied and given misleading information. Whether or not this is acceptable is a source of constant debate. The argument is usually that 'Many patients don't want to know the truth, even if they seemingly ask for it. It is therefore grossly irresponsible of us to tell them' *or* 'even if we tell them, they get the wrong end of the stick and end up worrying needlessly.' The issue is not, however, the crude one of 'To tell or not to tell'. It is rather, 'How do we tell them, at a level they can understand without distortion and at a pace at which they can accept it?' It is quite possible, though not easy or pleasant, to ascertain whether or not patients really want to know, whether they have understood and how they have accepted it (or not). It may not always be appropriate for the nurse who gave the information to check out the patient's understanding, especially if she/he is upset. However, another nurse could return later on to establish what the patient 'heard'. Being able to detect the 'faults' in giving information is a skill that is explored in Exercise 6.6.

Exercise 6.6   Deficiencies in giving information

Instructions

Please read the following explanation. Your task is to detect deficiencies in the way in which it is given. With a coloured pen underline each 'deficiency' and write in the right-hand column the nature of the deficiency.

Answer sheet

Staff nurse giving pre-operative information to   *Nature of deficiency*
female patient about to undergo a
cholecystectomy:

Tomorrow you're going to theatre. When
you come round you'll have an I.V. infusion
— nothing to worry about, it's just a drip.
So, the operation that you're having is a
cholecystectomy — that is, the removal of
your gall bladder, which is probably full of
stones. They may then explore the common
bile duct, which is a tube — a bit like a
drainpipe — which takes bile from the liver
to the gut. If the drainpipe is blocked, the
bile will spill over into the blood. Before
you go, we'll give you a pre-med., which
will make you fall asleep. When you come
back from theatre you'll have the drip, like I
said, and possibly a T -tube in the bile duct.
You'll also have a stab drain under your
ribs. When you come round you won't have
any more of that pain. You'll be fine, you'll
see. Of course, you'll be in for a bit before
you go. We'll be taking out alternate sutures
— probably on the 7th/8th day.

With a partner who has also completed the exercise, if possible, consider the discussion issues.

Discussion issues

1. What difficulties are there in detecting faults of information giving?
2. When might this skill be required in nursing settings?
3. What barriers do different nursing settings construct that make it difficult to improve upon information that has been given badly?

Comments

Questioning and giving information are both skills that can be employed in the pursuit of social goals, and have been discussed here in the context of 'control'. A further set of skills to be used in the realization of social goals are those concerned with assertiveness.

6.2 Assertiveness

Assertiveness is a particular form of control, and interest in it, as a specific skill, has grown in recent years. It is often thought that assertion is the skill of standing up for yourself and getting exactly what you want, either directly or by manipulating other people. Inherent in this notion is the exercise of power over other people. Assertion is not about power: it is better described as the *art of confident, clear, honest and direct communication, whilst at all times retaining respect for other people*. Assertiveness is non-aggressive, non-defensive and non-manipulative, and it does not interfere with other people's freedom to take an assertive stance or make appropriate decisions. To be assertive is not always to get our own way. It may well be that we reach a compromise on all/any of the issues(s). In reaching this position though, on being assertive, we should never compromise our own self-worth. All those involved should continue to feel acknowledged and not 'put down' or humiliated. If they do not feel acknowledged, it is likely that the encounter will have been handled aggressively or manipulatively, rather than assertively. A comparison of assertion, aggression, manipulation and passivity is made in Exercise 6.7.

Exercise 6.7 Assertion, aggression, passivity and manipulation

---

Instructions

Please think of a situation that occured during the last week that you would like to have handled more assertively. Outline this situation by completing the chart below.

Answer sheet

1. Which assertive right (see Table 6.3) arose in this situation?

2. Briefly describe what happened and how you handled the situation (aggressively/passively/manipulatively)

3. What could you have done to handle it more assertively?

With a partner who has also completed the exercise if possible, consider the discussion issues.

Discussion issues

1. Which style response do you use most frequently? Why?
2. Does your style of response vary between work and home? Why?
3. Do other people make it easy to be assertive? How/how not?

Comments

If assertion is not about getting our own way, what is it about? Table 6.3 lists what are known as *assertive rights*. These are the basic rights we have as people, and assertion is the articulation of these rights. There may be some other 'rights' that we have not included, and space has been left in Table 6.3 for these to be added.

A criticism that is often raised of this list is that to articulate all these rights would lead to selfishness and a lack of consideration for others. The important things to remember are:

(a)   One person's rights are *never* at the expense of another's. Everyone must be respected at all times.
(b)   What a person does should always be based on her/his assessment of what she/he wants to do, and she/he should not be prevented from making such an appraisal. What she/he *actually does* is her/his own decision, and as such should not be judged by others.

Most of us experience some difficulty in handling those interpersonal situations that require us to assert ourselves in some way. Examples of these might be turning down a request, asking a favour, accepting/giving a compliment, expressing approval/disapproval, accepting legitimate criticism or stating our preference. Exercise 6.8 provides the opportunity to reflect upon our own ease and difficulty in assertion.

Some basic assertive techniques

There are three components to the skill of assertion, and these are:

(a)   To be able to decide what it is you want or feel, and say so specifically and directly.
(b)   To stick to your statement, repeating it, if necessary, over and over again.
(c)   To deflect assertively any responses from the other person which might undermine your assertive stance.

Being specific

This is not as easy as it sounds. It means deciding what the point is and stating it without all the unnecessary padding we tend to use when we are uncomfortable or anxious. The nurse who seeks to 'soften the blow' when she/he tells a patient with whom she has a special relationship that she/he is moving wards, may say something like 'I know you'll be upset ... but don't

Table 6.3   Assertive rights

Assertiveness is seen to be the articulation of basic rights we have as people, and these are summarized below:

1. I have the right to state my own needs and set my own priorities as a person independent of any roles that I assume in my life.
2. I have the right to offer no reasons or excuses for justifying my behaviour.
3. I have the right to decline responsibility for other people's problems.
4. I have the right to change my mind.
5. I have the right to make mistakes.
6. I have the right to say 'I don't know'.
7. I have the right to deal with others without being dependent on them for approval.
8. I have the right to be illogical in making decisions.
9. I have the right to say 'I don't understand'.
10. I have the right to ask for what I want.
11. I have the right to say 'Yes' or 'No' for myself.
12. I have the right to express my feelings.
13. I have the right to express my opinions and values.
14. I have the right to be treated with respect as an intelligent, capable and equal human being.

Are there any other 'rights' you would like to add? If so, write them in.

15. ...
16. ...
17. ...
18. *I have the right to say 'No' without feeling guilty.*

Source: Adapted from M.J. Smith, *When I Say 'No', I Feel Guilty*, Bantam, New York, 1975

Exercise 6.8   Levels of assertion

Instructions

Please indicate your degree of discomfort or anxiety in the space provided *before* each situation listed below. Use the following scale to indicate degree of discomfort: 1 = none; 2 = a little; 3 = a fair amount; 4 = a lot; 5 = a great deal

Answer sheet

Degree of discomfort	*Situation*
_____	1. Turn down a request to borrow some of your clothes.
_____	2. Compliment a friend.
_____	3. Ask a favour of someone.
_____	4. Decline to answer personal questions.
_____	5. Apologize when you are at fault.
_____	6. Turn down a request for a meeting.
_____	7. Admit fear or anxiety and ask that allowances be made.
_____	8. Tell a person you are intimately involved with when she/he says or does something that bothers you.
_____	9. Ask for an increase in pay.
_____	10. Admit ignorance in some area.
_____	11. Turn down a request to spend time with someone.
_____	12. Ask personal questions.
_____	13. Stop a talkative friend.
_____	14. Initiate a conversation with a stranger.
_____	15. Compliment a person you are romantically involved with.
_____	16. Your initial request for a meeting is turned down and you ask the person again at a later date.
_____	17. Admit confusion about a point under discussion at work.
_____	18. Apply for a job.
_____	19. Ask whether you have offended someone.
_____	20. Tell someone that you like her/him.
_____	21. Request expected service when such is not forthcoming, for example, in a restaurant.
_____	22. Tell someone when you think you have been belittled.

_____	23.	Return defective items, for example, to a shop.
_____	24.	Express an opinion that differs from that of a (senior) person you are talking to.
_____	25.	Resist sexual advances when you are not interested.
_____	26.	Tell the person when she/he has done something that is unfair to you.
_____	27.	Tell someone good news about yourself.
_____	28.	Resist pressure to drink.
_____	29.	Resist a significant person's unfair demand.
_____	30.	Leave a job.
_____	31.	Discuss openly with the person her/his criticism of your work.
_____	32.	Request the return of borrowed items.
_____	33.	Receive compliments.
_____	34.	Continue to talk to someone who disagrees with you.
_____	35.	Tell a friend or someone you work with when she/he says or does something that irritates you.
_____	36.	Ask a person who is annoying you in a public place to stop (for example, smoking, radio turned on too loud, etc.)

Now, please indicate the situations you would like to handle more assertively by placing a circle around the item number.

Source: Adapted from E.D. Gambrill and C.A. Richey (1975) An assertion inventory for use in assessment and research, *Behaviour Therapy*, Vol. 6, pp 550–61

When you have completed the questionnaire, consider the discussion issues.

Discussion issues

1. How do we learn to be assertive or not?
2. Does your training in nursing encourage you to be assertive?
3. Are you more assertive in some situations than others? Why do you think this is?
4. Are there any situations at work where you would never consider being assertive? Please describe. Why do you think this is?

Comments

worry, I'll come and visit you ... the thing is ... I won't be coming on this ward again.' The trouble with padding is that it often weakens the statement and confuses the listener (which may be what is intended!).

Exercise 6.9 offers the opportunity to practise being specific.

It is only possible to be specific when we are clear about what it is we *want* to say. Once we know this, the task is to be able to say clearly and directly what we want or feel. It is rarely sufficient to rely on hints and innuendo, assuming that the other person should know what we want. This simply gives the other person the opportunity at a later date to accuse us of never really asking. (The 'why didn't you say so' phenomenon, when we though we had!)

Clarity and directness is often confused with bluntness or rudeness, and in efforts to avoid making others feel guilty or uncomfortable we learn to avoid such directness. We often resort, instead, to complaint, reproach, sarcasm and sulkiness. Ironically, these strategies often 'work' by making the other person feel guilty!

Sticking to it

This means learning to be persistent, and to behave as if we were a record that had got stuck (this technique is sometimes referred to as the 'Broken Record'). The purpose of repetition is to help maintain a steady position without being sidetracked by irrelevant, manipulative or argumentative comments from the other person. Other people will often try to divert us from the point we are trying to make by asking subsidiary questions: as soon as we reply to these we are hooked, and our position is weakened.

Consider the patient who is on a reducing diet. The patient is about to tuck into the jam sponge and custard when the nurse reminds her/him of her/his diet. Then ...

(a) *Patient:*   You're not really interested in my well-being, are you?
   Loser reply: Of course I am ...
   Persistent reply: I know you like it, but you are not allowed jam sponge and custard.
(b) *Patient:*   The trouble is, you don't understand about my diet do you?
   Loser reply: Yes I do. It's carefully planned.
   Persistent reply: It's hard and I know you hate it, but you're not to eat jam sponge and custard.

Exercise 6.9   Being specific

Instructions

In each of the following examples, please underline the point of the statement and put the padding in brackets. For example:

(I hope you don't think I'm being rude ... I wouldn't normally say anything, but ...) <u>your zip is undone.</u>

Answer sheet

1. I'm terribly sorry to trouble you but I wonder if you'd mind ... I mean, could I have a bedpan?
2. Oh, I'd have loved to have helped, if only you'd asked me earlier, but with things as they are, I'm awfully busy, so I'm sorry, but I can't.
3. I expect you'll think I'm rather forward ... I don't know you very well ... but I do think your hair is lovely.
4. My mother always said I'm not much of a judge of character, but I'd say you were an understanding sort of a person.
5. I know it's late and you're probably full up, but if it's possible and you can manage it, I'd like to make an appointment for this morning: if you can manage to fit me in, I'd be very grateful.

When you have completed the examples, consider the Discussion Issues.

Discussion issues

1. What characterizes situations where specificity is difficult to achieve (that is role/relative ages/intimacy etc.)?
2. Why does padding occur in times of anxiety? What functions does sit serve?

Comments

In this example, the nurse has refused to be deflected from her/his statements that the patient should not eat the pudding despite attempts to engage her/him in discussions of concern for patients or dietary knowledge.

Repeating a phrase endlessly, albeit in different forms, may lead to an aggressive outburst or sulky submission, as either the person who is trying to be assertive gets sidetracked or she/he is unable to respond appropriately to the other person's deflections. With practice, though, we should be able to 'stick to a point' more firmly, and without unpleasant consequences.

Fielding responses

This is the ability to indicate we have heard what another person has said, without getting 'hooked' by what she/he has said. Consider the following:

> You may have been able to walk to X-ray before, but *today you are to go in a chair.*
>
> I know that you want to use the telephone, but *I need to use it myself right now.*
>
> I appreciate that you have covered for me in the past, but *I can't work late tonight.*
>
> I can see that you are feeling let down, but *I cannot give you another pain killer.*

'Broken Record' and fielding responses are examined in Exercise 6.10.

We mentioned above that assertiveness often results in both parties reaching a workable compromise. If both partners have strong commitments to their positions, the outcome is more likely to be a compromise (though never at the expense of loss of self-worth or respect). Suppose, for instance, that a ward sister who was short staffed, needed the staff nurse to work a weekend she/he was due to have off, and the staff nurse had prior engagements. Acceptable compromises might be for the staff nurse to work some of the weekend, fitting in her/his prior engagements *or* to have some other (desirable) time off in lieu. There are many instances daily when the most assertive action is to achieve a satisfactory compromise, instead of adopting a stubborn, selfish and insensitive stance.

Exercise 6.10   Broken record and fielding responses

Instructions

In groups of three, allocate the roles A, B and C. Read the following instructions for each role.

1. A — *assertive person*. Choose a situation that you would like to handle more assertively (use Exercise 6.8 to identify this situation if you like). Describe a typical instance to B. Give B a 'role' to play as you partner in the situation. Tell B how to behave. Act out the scene and try to be as assertive as possible.

2. B — *partner, intent on sidetracking A*. Play the role that A has described. Try to ensure that A's attempts to be assertive fail. Try to sidetrack A.

3. C — 'coach'. Watch what happens when A and B act out the scene. Note when you think A could have been more assertive, or when she/he succumbed to B's diversions. Take notes if appropriate. At the end of the role play 'coach' A in how she/he could have been more assertive or have avoided B's diversions by using the broken record. If B was not good at diverting, do you have any suggestions as to how she/he could have been more effective?

4. Act out the role play. Discuss fully what happened, and how each person felt in her/his role. Do this for fifteen minutes. Swop roles and repeat. Swop roles again, and repeat.

5. Repeat exercise with C 'coaching' for the skills of '*fielding responses*'. At the end of the exercise, discuss with each other some of the consequences of fielding responses. Refer to the text if you are unsure of the skills of broken record and fielding responses.

6. When you have completed all the role plays, consider the discussion issues.

Discussion issues

1. What characterizes situations where it is difficult to use the skills of broken record and fielding responses?

2. Are there any situations at work in which you find it particularly difficult to use the skills of broken record and/or fielding responses?

3. Can you think of any people who are particularly good at preventing you using the skills of broken record and/or fielding responses? What are they like? (That is what relationship do you have with them — relatives, subordinate, superior, friend, stranger, etc.)

4. What difficulties did you have role playing these skills? Why was this?

Comments

Handling criticism

Once we have acquired the basic skills of assertion, we can begin to think of applying them to familiar situations. Being criticized is, perhaps the inter-personal event that most frequently leaves us feeling angry, hard-done-by and humiliated. When other people criticize us, they usually criticize something about us as people or about what we do. Criticism always contains an arbitrary right/wrong value judgement which often goes unrealized as the critics assume that everyone would share their assessment of what is right or wrong. So, to tell someone 'All those late nights have made you late again' is to imply that they are naughty/irresponsible/inappropriately fond of the high-life, etc. In other words, that being late is wrong, and this is due to the late nights, which are also wrong. Some aspects of criticisms may well be justified, but some may be unjustified, implying all sorts of hidden meanings. The assertive way to deal with criticism is to confront both these aspects: to acknowledge those parts that are justified and to challenge those that are not. Consider the following:

(a) *Sister:* All those late nights have made you late again.
     Nurse: I'm sorry I'm late. (*Justified criticism.*) I'll try to get here on time in the future. (*Avoiding provocation.*)
(b) *Patient 1:* I really do think you are a cold, unfeeling person.
     Patient 2: You may be right. (*Justified criticism.*) I've never made friends easily. (*Explanation.*)

Both these respondents acknowledged the truths that were contained in the criticism, and thus avoided acting defensively as, for example:

(a) *Nurse:* I'm not usually late, not like some people. (*Defensive.*)
(b) *Patient 2:* Other people don't think so. (*Defensive, critical.*)

In these examples, the respondent, whilst acknowledging legitimate criticism gave passive replies that might encourage the speaker to pursue her/his criticism. A different way to deal assertively with criticism is to challenge the basis of the right-wrong judgements made by the critic. By being asked for clarification or expansion, the critics are encouraged to examine their own right-wrong judgements, and to state more clearly and honestly what they are feeling. In other words, they are given the chance to act more assertively themselves. Consider, for example, the following:

(a) *Nurse 1:* You are always flying off the handle.
   Nurse 2: When do I fly off the handle? (*Request for clarification.*)
(b) *Nurse:* You are always sitting around reading the paper.
   Patient: I do like to read the paper as soon as possible (*Justified criticism.*)
   What is it about reading the paper that is bad? (*Request for expansion.*).
(c) *Sister:* Haven't you done this yet?
   . *Nurse:* No. (*Justified criticism.*) When did you want it done by? (*Request for expansion.*)
(d) *Student 1:* We should cooperate more, so we can get it done more easily.
   Student 2: How can we be more cooperative? (*Request for clarification/expansion.*)

Our skills of handling criticism are challenged in Exercise 6.11.

Handling compliments

Exercise 6.11 is about dealing with (justified) criticism. Interestingly, giving and receiving compliments assertively is often felt to be more difficult than dealing with criticism. Compliments, too, generally contain a component that is justified and an arbitrary value judgement, although in this case the value is usually positive. Compliments may be handled in much the same way as criticisms are. Take, for example, a doctor telling a nurse 'The way you handled her panic attack was very helpful.' Such a comment invites different responses

(a) Thank you, I tried to remember what I had been taught.
(b) Thank you: how exactly was it helpful?
(c) What makes you think it might not have been?

We can see from these replies that the compliment can be taken in good grace; used as the basis for discussion; or denied, and treated defensively as if it were a criticism.

Exercise 6.11   Dealing with criticism

Instructions

Section A

Can you give some assertive replies to the following criticisms?

Criticism   *Assertive reply*

1. I'd appreciate it if you didn't send
   someone along for the blood at the
   last minute.
2. Haven't you sorted those samples
   yet?
3. You simply make work for yourself,
   taking notes like that.
4. Have you got other shoes to wear
   with your uniform?

Section B

Now think of three recent examples of instances where you were criticized. Write down the criticism. What did you say? What could you have said to be assertive?

Criticism   *What did you say?*   *Assertive reply*

1.
2.
3.

With a partner, who has also completed this exercise if possible, consider the discussion issues.

Discussion issues

1. Is criticism more difficult to deal with assertively in particular relationships?
2. Does role impinge upon the ability to deal with criticisms assertively?
3. Does this exercise help you think of ways that criticism can be constructive? Give examples.

Comments

Exercise 6.12   Receiving and giving compliments

Instructions

Section A

Can you give some assertive replies to the following compliments?

Compliment   *Assertive reply*

1. You are looking well.
2. You seem to get a lot done in a
    morning.
3. Those colours suit you.
4. I've never had blood taken so
    painlessly.

Section B

In pairs, take it in turns to compliment your partner about

(a)   her/his looks
(b)   her/his behaviour
(c)   her/his characteristics ('nature')

What did you feel about doing this? Why?

(a)

(b)

(c)

Discuss these feelings with your partner.

With a partner who has also completed this exercise if possible, consider the discussion issues.

Discussion issues

1. What factors make it easy or hard to receive compliments assertively?
2. What factors make it easy/hard to give compliments assertively?
3. Would the task in Section B have been easier/harder with someone you knew less well/better/older/younger etc.?
4. Are compliments easier to give/accept at home or work? Why?

Comments

We do have a tendency to deny compliments, to react as though the person offering the compliment was being sarcastic or even rude. In other words we assume a latent meaning to what she/he said (see Section 3.2). However, if we are to assume that everyone should be enabled to act assertively, then, given the definition of assertion as honest and direct communication, we must take compliments on their face value not in terms of their latent meaning.

Having said this though, we are generally well used to using compliments as a means of being sarcastic. On the whole people find it as hard to give genuine compliments as to receive them. For some reason we find the expression of positive feelings towards others as (if not more) difficult as negative ones. Exercise 6.12 offers the opportunity to examine this difficulty.

In Exercises 6.7–6.12 some assertion skills have been introduced. They are skills and will only come easily with practice. As nurses, though, every day provides lots of opportunities to practise them, and it is possible for us all, individually, to monitor our levels of assertion by completing the questionnaire in Exercise 6.8 at regular intervals.

We have discussed above three of the most common sources of difficulty with assertion, namely handling criticism and giving and receiving compliments. There are other, perhaps more complex assertive skills that nurses require in order to exercise control in their interpersonal lives. We discuss persuasion and attitude change (Chapter 7), and counselling (Chapter 8) elsewhere.

6.3 Summary

This chapter has been concerned with basic skills of control in personal encounters, namely the use of questions, giving information and explanation and assertiveness. Specifically, the following issues were raised:

Control is central to all interpersonal relationships, and ranges from subtle influence to deliberate regulation of others.

Questioning, instructing, explaining and reassuring are frequent forms of control for nurses.

Questioning serves to elicit information and to encourage a person to explore a range of experiences.

Questions serve many different social functions, in different situations.

Questions, as part of social rituals, may be ambiguous.

Appropriate style of questioning is determined by the situation and the questioner's goals.

Depending on the situation, open and closed questions might be helpful.

Leading, multiple and rhetorical questions are rarely helpful.

Information and reassurance are often confused.

Patients' needs should be assessed prior to giving information/explanation.

Giving information involves stages of establishing needs, checking, planning, presenting and concluding.

The presentation of information requires decisions to be made regarding the issue(s), elaboration(s), checking understanding and clarification.

Insufficient attention to how information is given may lead to inaccuracy.

Assertiveness is the art of confident, clear, honest and direct communication whilst at all times retaining respect for other people.

Assertion can be distinguished from passivity, aggression and manipulation.

Assertion frequently involves reaching a compromise.

'Assertive rights' underlie the need to develop skills of assertion.

Basic assertive techniques include being specific, sticking to the point, and deflecting attempts at sidetracking.

Handling criticism, and giving/receiving compliments are sources of difficulty in assertion for many people.

Further reading

Davis, B. (1985) The clinical effects of interpersonal skills. In C. Kagan (Ed.)
    Interpersonal Skills in Nursing: Research and Applications, Croom Helm, London
Dickson, A. (1982) *A Woman in Your Own Right: Assertiveness and You*, Quartet
    Books, London
Faulknder, A. (1984) Communication of information to patients. In A. Faulkner (Ed.)
    Recent Advances in Nursing, Communication, Churchill Livingstone, Edinburgh
French, P. (1983) Explanation, questioning and interviewing, *Social Skills and
    Nursing Practice*, Croom Helm, London, ch. 4
Smith, M.J. (1975) *When I say No I Feel Guilty*, Bantam, New York
Wilson-Barnett, J. (1981) Communicating with patients in general wards. In W. Bridge
    and J. Macleod Clark, *Communication in Nursing Care*, H.M. and M., Aylesbury

CHAPTER 7

SOCIAL PROBLEM SOLVING

We have seen, in Chapters 5 and 6, that facilitation and assertion skills are essential to many interpersonal situations. If we are to use these skills effectively, we have to be able to decide which to use in which situation. In other words, we have to think about what we want to achieve in a specific situation and choose an appropriate strategy. The ability to perceive accurately social cues and decide upon suitable social action is itself a skill, albeit a *cognitive* skill rather than a *performance* one. In this chapter we shall look at some cognitive aspects of interaction. We will concentrate on social problem solving, with specific reference to the nature of attitudes and prejudice and attempts to change them.

7.1 The social problem solving process

Many interpersonal situations require that we think carefully of how we are going to handle them. In doing this, firstly we need to identify precisely what it is about the situation that is difficult or problematic. Following this, we need to think about alternative ways we could act and what the effects of these might be. Then, having chosen a course of action we have to follow it, and finally attempt to assess whether we have, in fact, dealt with the problem effectively. Figure 7.1 summarizes the stages of social problem solving. Let us see how this process relates to a real situation.

Figure 7.1   The social problem solving process

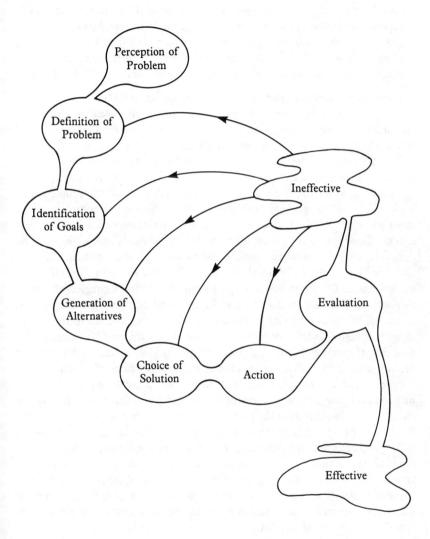

Consider the following:

Female medical ward in large city general hospital. It is evening. Seven patients are in the day room after visitors have left. Two Asian women are eating curried snacks brought to them by their visitors. The third Asian woman turns the TV on. A young white woman begins shouting (racial) abuse at the Asian women which attracts the attention of the ward sister.

What should she do? And how should she go about it?

Perception of the situation: The sister must notice that something is amiss and make judgements, from what she can see/hear, as to what is going on. As a result, she must *define the problem*. In the example, she may pick up what is being said, and consider the problem to be either a dispute over choice of TV programme, or a dislike of curry smells. On the other hand, she may consider the problem to be one of racial conflict. Her definition of the problem will lead her to think of possible outcomes or *goals*. She may, therefore, consider *either* a compromise over TV programmes, *or* the Asian women eating their snacks elsewhere *or* a challenge to the white woman's racist views to be desirable goals, depending on her formulation of the problem. Having identified her goals, she must then consider *various strategies* she can use to achieve them. Once she has generated some alternative strategies, she must *choose* those that she thinks likely to be the most effective and then *act* on them. All the time she must be *evaluating* this course of action to see if it is, indeed, effective. If it is not, she can do one of four things: (1) reconsider the problem; (2) change her objectives or goals; (3) look at some more ways of dealing with the situation; or (4) choose a different course of action.

From the moment she notices the disturbance, the sister must run through, in her mind, the different stages of social problem solving, and as a result change her behaviour until the problem is 'solved' to her satisfaction. Clearly, the better able she is at doing this, the more effective she is likely to be.

The skills that are part of social problem solving ability are, then, *perception of social cues*, accuracy in *identifying own and others' goals*, *capacity to generate alternative strategies* and the *insight to judge the effectiveness* of chosen strategies. We have explored elsewhere (see Chapter 3) the perception of social cues. Exercise 7.1 is concerned with the identification of social goals and the generation of alternative strategies for achieving them.

The social problem solving approach can be applied to any situation. It is not always as conscious as we have implied here: some people naturally adopt a problem solving approach to various social situations. Indeed, it has been suggested that problem solving ability distinguishes those who are rigid and

Exercise 7.1   Identification of goals and alternative strategies

---

Instructions

Watch a film of some nursing activities. (For example, from the 'Communication in Patient Care' series, see Appendix III or a sample from a soap opera from TV.) Watch the scene and complete the answer sheet below.

Answer sheet

Can you identify the *goals* of the nurse in this scene? (i.e. what was she/he trying to do?)

What *alternative strategies* could she/he have used to achieve this goal?

Main goal(s)

1.
2.
3.

Sub-goal(s)

1.
2.
3.

Consider, with a partner who has also completed the task if possible, the discussion issues.

Discussion issues

1. Did the context affect the judgement of the actors' goals? How?
2. Would the goals have been different if the actors were (a) different nationalities, (b) younger, (c) the opposite sex? If so, why?
3. If the interaction had taken place elsewhere, would you have been able to think of more alternative strategies?
4. What features of the context limited the choice of alternatives for the actors?

Comments

relatively poor at dealing with interpersonal situations from those who are flexible and relatively adept at dealing with them. It follows then, that practice in social problem solving skills may lead to more effective interpersonal functioning. Exercise 7.2 gives some practice in using the social problem solving process.

The example given in Exercise 7.2 is an interesting one in so far as it not only concerns people's behaviour, but also their attitudes — in this case their racist attitudes. As attitudes underlie a great deal of our interpersonal behaviour, and as nurses often have to try to get people to change their attitudes in one way or another, we will take some time now to discuss them.

7.2 Attitudes

Attitudes do not exist as such. So how do we know what a person's attitudes are? Generally, we look at their behaviour and infer their attitudes from the way they behave. Similarly, it can be argued that we infer our own attitudes from seeing how we ourselves behave. One of the reasons we make judgements about other people's attitudes is so that we can make predictions about how they behave. Whilst this might appear sensible and a useful way of organizing a lot of information about others, it can lead us into difficulties as people do not always behave in accordance with their (assumed) attitudes.

The nature of attitudes

It can be useful to think of three parts of an attitude, as illustrated in Figure 7.2. Firstly there is the *cognitive or thinking* part, for example, 'I think men and women are equally suited to nursing.' Then there is the *affective or feeling* part, for example, 'I feel angry when men are refused places on nurse training courses.' And finally there is the *conative or action* part, for example, 'I encourage men and women to apply for nurse training and do all I can to select suitable applicants whether they be men or women.' Generally it is assumed that the three parts of an attitude are consistent, but this is not always so, and, as we shall see later, the inconsistency between parts of an attitude may be exploited in attempts to change attitudes.

Exercise 7.2   Social problem solving

Instructions

With reference to Figure 7.1, please consider how you would deal with the following situations using a social problem solving approach.

Answer sheet

1. *Problem:* Coronary care unit in district general hospital. Middle-aged man readmitted with suspected myocardial infarction, 6 hours previously. On talking to you, a third-year student nurse, he becomes verbally abusive and agitated. He complains that the doctor(s) have given him no information and that senior medical personnel have not visited him, that the ward is noisy, that the bed is uncomfortable, that the lights are too bright, and that nurses' lack of concern is reflected in their refusal to allow him visitors. Makes attempts to get out of bed, threatening that he is going home.

How would you deal with this problem?

2. *Problem:* Male orthopaedic ward. 21-year-old man admitted following motor cycle accident with fractured shaft of femur. You are a student nurse in charge of ward whilst sister is on her meal break during evening visiting. Man's mother, who is herself a senior nurse tutor, queries the proposed plan of treatment. Your answer is unsatisfactory, and the mother demands to see someone more senior. You are unable to arrange this. The mother then states that she will contact the Director of Nursing Services to complain about your attitude.

How would you deal with this problem?

3. Now, please think of a problem you have met at work recently. Outline the problem and indicate how you might deal with it using a social problem solving approach.

Problem:

How would you deal with this problem?

Consider your answers in the light of the discussion issues.

Discussion issues

1. Are any of the stages of the problem solving process more difficult than others?
2. How would the problem solving process differ if you had full responsibility for the situation?
3. What barriers to effective social problem solving are there in nursing?
4. Could the social problem solving process be used by patients?

Comments

Figure 7.2   The nature of attitudes

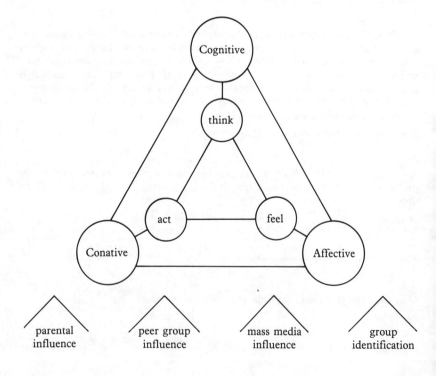

So far, then, we have argued that attitudes are 'hypothetical constructs' in that they are inferred (sometimes inaccurately) from behaviour. It can be useful to think about the thinking, feeling and action parts of an attitude and the extent to which they are consistent with each other. Attitudes help us to make predictions about how we and others will behave and to express values about objects, events or people. As we can see from Figure 7.2 attitudes develop as a response to various influences, including parental/family, peer group, mass media or group identity influences. In other words attitudes develop as part of the general process of socialization, and Exercise 7.3 allows us to explore the origins of some of our own attitudes.

Sometimes attitudes can be particularly strong and lead us to have biased predictions about other people's behaviour. Such strong attitudes are known as prejudices, and if acted upon may amount to discrimination.

Prejudice

We are all prejudiced about some things, events or people, and Exercise 7.4 is an exploration of the meaning of prejudice.

Our prejudices are frequently based on stereotypes, are emotionally charged, and if they are expressed, take the form of discrimination. As such they have unpleasant interpersonal consequences. Unfortunately, prejudices are usually faulty, inflexible and difficult to change. One of the pre-requisites for prejudice is that a person or an object can be seen to be different (and then discriminated against). This is one reason why racial prejudice is often linked with colour. In nursing there are many opportunities to see other people as different: opportunities that are often linked with different illnesses or disabilities. Obvious examples are where there are clear signs, and illness is easily detected. People with Parkinsons disease, facial palsy, scar tissue on face or hands, varying degrees of paralysis or spasticity, and those who are over/under weight may all appear different, and thus be the objects of prejudice. People with mental and physical handicaps, too, may be discriminated against as might those with degenerative diseases such as multiple sclerosis, motor neurone disease, etc. People who need prostheses of one sort or another, ranging from glasses, hearing aids, tooth braces and neck supports to artificial limbs and aids such as sticks, frames or wheelchairs can all be identified and stand in danger of being prejudiced against. The idea is that they are burdened with a characteristic that brands them as different —

Exercise 7.3   The development of attitudes

Instructions

Please think of two attitudes that you hold towards work, sex, sports, and discipline. Write one attitude in each of the rectangular boxes. Then think how this attitude has come about, and draw lines to those socializing agents that have influenced you. On each line, write how you were influenced.

EXAMPLE
WORK

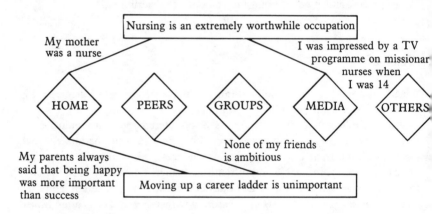

Answer sheet

WORK

HOME   PEERS   GROUPS   MEDIA   OTHERS?

SEX

HOME   PEERS   GROUPS   MEDIA   OTHERS?

SPORTS

HOME   PEERS   GROUPS   MEDIA   OTHERS?

DISCIPLINE

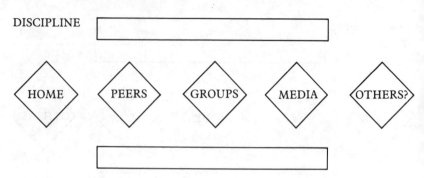

Look at your completed answer sheet and consider the discussion issues.

Discussion issues

1. Is it more difficult to see where some attitudes have come from than others? Why?
2. Which socializing agent has been the most important for the development of your attitudes?
3. Have you ever influenced anyone else's attitudes? What was this like?

Comments

Exercise 7.4   The meaning of prejudice

Instructions

Please think about the meaning of the word *prejudice*. Think about the development, nature and possibilities for changing prejudices, as well as your own prejudices. On the diagram below, write a label or a statement on each 'spike' of the circle, reflecting the particular segment of meaning. When complete, consider the discussion issues with a partner who has also completed the exercise if possible.

Answer sheet

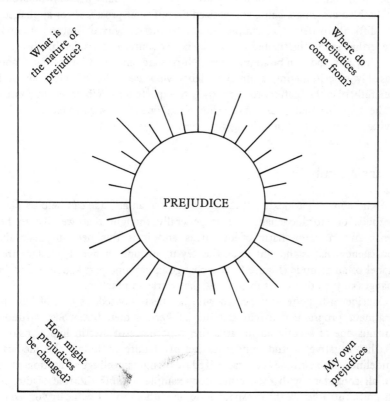

What is the nature of prejudice?

Where do prejudices come from?

PREJUDICE

How might prejudices be changed?

My own prejudices

Discussion issues

1. What is the function of prejudice?
2. Why are only certain individuals/groups the objects of prejudice?
3. Why do individuals vary in the amount of prejudice they display?
4. What is it about nursing that makes prejudice likely/unlikely to occur?
5. How important is membership of, and identification with, specific groups in the propagation of prejudice?

Comments

and often bad: in other words they are stigmatized. Many people who are ill or disabled anticipate being stigmatized even if their prostheses or appliances are difficult to detect. (Examples might be mastectomy or stoma patients). Nevertheless the anticipated stigma can be the source of considerable distress.

Behaviour, too, can be stigmatizing. Nurses are renowned for disliking (and possibly discriminating against) patients who ask a lot of questions and generally play the 'patient role' contrary to expectations. Whatever the source of the prejudice that results in discrimination, one of the ways to tackle it is by trying to change the underlying attitudes.

Changing attitudes

We said above that looking at the three parts of an attitude can help us plan methods of attitude change. It is generally thought that we like to be consistent in many parts of our lives and it is this need to maintain consistency that is thought to be the key to attitude change. If we take the model of an attitude (Figure 7.2), a change in any one part should result in changes in the others. Let us see how that works in practice.

Consider a hypertensive person who has been advised, as part of her/his treatment programme to cut salt out of her/his diet, but whose attitude remains one of scepticism towards the importance of diet in hypertension. Her/his negative attitude underlies her/his failure to follow the medical guidelines. The attitude is characterized by thoughts, feelings and actions that are all consistent with each other (for example, I *think* the role of diet is insignificant: I *dislike* the prospect of doing without salt: I will carry on *using* salt). If we were able to create some inconsistency within this system, the attitude may change. So, for example, giving the patient information may change her/his thoughts:

> It seems the role of diet *is* significant, so I'll stop using salt and maybe it won't be so bad. (*Change of attitude.*)

Alternatively, having the person in hospital may afford the chance to make her/him stop using salt, with a consequent change in the other components (hospital catering facilities permitting!)

> I have been forced to stop using salt, so there must be something in the link between diet and high blood pressure so I feel better about it. (*Change of attitude.*)

There are several different ways an attitude change can come about in whole or in part, and we've illustrated only two. However, the principle remains — disrupt the consistency (or congruence or consonance as it is sometimes called) between components of an attitude and this will lead us to experience tension (or inconsistency, incongruence or dissonance) which we then try to remove by changing the other parts accordingly. This tension is called cognitive dissonance: it is thought to be unpleasant, and as a result we do all we can do to reduce it. Of course, we may simply rationalize the change in the first part of the attitude (for example, the information I've been given is unreliable: hospital dieticians are unnecessarily ruthless, etc.), in which case no attitude change will follow. Exercise 7.5 is an examination of ways of reducing cognitive dissonance. The skill is to choose those ploys that will increase the likelihood of attitude change. Exercise 7.5 is essentially one example of social problem solving skill, namely the skill of persuasion.

7.3 Persuasion

There are many situations where nurses have to persuade other people to do something. They may have to persuade patients about the advisability of doing certain things connected with their illness and/or treatment, or colleagues to cooperate in some way. The issue will vary from those that nurses have little commitment to, to those that they feel deeply concerned about. Whatever the issue though, persuasion must be planned, and the social problem solving process outlined above is a useful framework for thinking about effective persuasion (see Figure 7.1).

Effective persuasive appeals

In addition to the phases of social problem solving, three other factors must also be considered. Firstly, the *source* of the persuasive appeal will affect how readily it is absorbed; so, conveying who it is that authorizes the message will influence its strength. Let us take various attempts to get people to change diet, or activities in the name of health education. If second-year student nurses were to endorse, say, the importance of taking more exercise for physical well-being, they would have little impact. If, however, senior physicians (in white coats!) or top sports personalities endorse the message, it may well have greater impact for certain groups. Thus the credibility, popularity and trustworthiness of the persuader should be considered.

Exercise 7.5   Cognitive dissonance and attitude change

Instructions

Familiarize yourself with the concept of cognitive dissonance. Please try to think of examples of attempts to reduce cognitive dissonance and the strategies used to reduce it. Complete the chart below.

Example

Cognitive dissonance
I am overweight and yet I know this exacerbates my arthritis.

Dissonance-reducing strategy
Change: I will go on a diet.
Repression: I will focus on the way the weather affects my arthritis.
Rationalization: I have always been overweight. *Or* Jean has arthritis and she is not overweight etc.
Belittling the dissonance: If my weight didn't bother me, something else would

Answer sheet

1. *Patients*
Cognitive dissonance   *Dissonance-reducing strategy*

2. *Colleagues*
Cognitive dissonance   *Dissonance-reducing strategy*

3. *Myself*
Cognitive dissonance   *Dissonance-making strategy*

Consider your answers with reference to the discussion issues.

Discussion issues

1. Are people who are ill more likely to use particular strategies for reducing dissonance?
2. Do high status people use particular strategies for reducing dissonance?
3. Do your own strategies for reducing dissonance vary with the situation/issue?

Comments

Secondly, *the nature of the communication* — the message itself and the medium through which it is sent — will influence its acceptability. The message may be emotional or fear producing and may or may not have specific recommendations for action. It may appeal to reason, presenting a one or two-sided argument; it may be humorous and entertaining; it may contain the essence of the message at the beginning, middle or end of the total communication and it may or may not take into account the present level of opinion. The message may be spoken, written, recorded, drawn, video taped or be in the form of a song or play, etc. Different messages to different audiences will require different types of persuasive appeals.

Finally, the *nature of the audience* or recipients of the communication must be considered. If people have had prior experience of attempts to be persuaded, they may have been 'inoculated' against the appeal, and thus react against further attempts at persuasion: furthermore, people with low self-esteem are more easily persuaded and vice versa. A group audience may react differently from individual(s) to different types of appeal. The factors to bear in mind when planning a persuasive message are summarized in Table. 7.1

In short, persuasion must take account of *who says what to whom via what medium and with what effect?* This last point is an important one as in order to gauge whether or not persuasion was effective, we should have some idea of what a desirable change would be (e.g. behaviour/attitude change etc.) Exercise 7.6 affords the opportunity to plan and execute a persuasive appeal that is of relevance to nurses.

Persuasion is often used in attempts to change attitudes and, in turn, to change behaviour. It can be argued that perhaps the greatest challenge to nurses is of how to effect changes in their patients that require their willingness and cooperation. Medical and nursing procedures cannot always be imposed upon patients, and the interpersonal aspects of these procedures require nurses to have considerable social problem solving skills.

Table 7.1   Factors influencing persuasive appeals

Source (Who?)

Credibility and expertise
Popularity (media/sports/pop stars, etc.)
Trustworthiness (related to triviality of issue)

Nature (How?)

1. Message:
   (a) Emotionally arousing/appealing to reason
   (b) One- or two-sided argument
   (c) Order of presentation
   (d) Present opinions of audience?

2. Channel:
   (a) visual
   (b) auditory
   (c) entertainment

Audience characteristics (to whom?)

Initial position
Level self-esteem
Group/individual(s)
Prior experience and 'inoculation'

Effects (What should change?)

Behaviour
Attitudes
Thoughts
Beliefs

Exercise 7.6   Persuasive appeals

Instructions

With two or three colleagues, if possible, prepare a persuasive appeal about one of the following issues:

Persuasive appeals
1. Please become a blood donor.
2. Do not smoke on wards which use oxygen.
3. Have your babies inoculated.
4. It is not a good idea to rely on tranquillizers.
5. People with mental handicaps have a right to an ordinary life.
6. Procedures for infection control on the wards must be followed.

   In planning your appeal, pay due consideration to the factors summarized in Table 7.1. The appeal can be for any channel and for any audience.

   Discuss the experience of generating this persuasive appeal with reference to the discussion issues.

Discussion issues

1. How would you evaluate whether the persuasive appeal had worked or not?
2. How often do nurses have to construct persuasive appeals? Give examples.
3. Have you ever been influenced by someone else's persuasive appeal? What did you find convincing about it?
4. Would your persuasive appeal have been different if the audience were older/younger, more/less informed etc.? In what ways?

Comments

7.4 Summary

This chapter has been concerned with social problem solving skills and their application in the context of attitude change and persuasion. Specifically the following issues were raised:

Cognitive aspects are as important as performance aspects of interpersonal skill.

Social problem solving ability is fundamental to effective interpersonal skill.

Perception of the situation leads to definition of the problem.

It is necessary to identify the goals or possible outcomes before engaging upon a course of action.

Appropriate strategies must be considered in pursuit of the identified goals.

When a strategy has been chosen, it must be carefully monitored and evaluated to see if it is having the desired effect.

On evaluating the effects of a particular strategy the options to change goals or reconsider alternatives should remain open.

The more flexible a person is with regard to social problem solving, the more interpersonally skilled she/he is likely to be.

The more rigid a person is with regard to social problem solving, the less interpersonally skilled she/he is likely to be.

Social problem solving is not always a conscious process, but at any time it can become so.

Attempting to change attitudes is a common social problem solving situation for nurses.

Attitudes do not exist, they are inferred.

Attitudes can be thought of in terms of cognitive, emotional and behavioural components.

A change in any one component of an attitude may result in changes in other components.

Inconsistency between parts of an attitude may lead to the experience of cognitive dissonance.

People attempt to reduce cognitive dissonance whenever they can.

Prejudice is a strong attitude and if acted upon may lead to discrimination.

Prejudice and discrimination are closely linked to stigma.

Stigma may be real or perceived.

Prejudice is difficult to change.

Persuasion is often used in attempts to change attitudes and/or behaviour.

The source, nature and medium of the message all influence persuasive appeals.

Audience characteristics influence persuasive appeals.

Persuasion is a particular form of social problem solving.

Further reading

Goffman, E. (1968) *Stigma. Notes on the Management of Spoiled Identity*, Penguin, Harmondsworth

Katz, J. (1978) *White Awareness*, University of Oklahoma Press, Norman, Oklahoma

Macmillan, P. (1983–4) Ward Management, series in *Nursing Times*

Reich, B. and Adcock, C. (1976) *Values, Attitudes and Behaviour Change*, Methuen, London

Roberts, D. Nonverbal communication, Popular and unpopular patients. In A. Faulkner (Ed.) *Recent Advances in Nursing, 7, Communication*, Churchill Livingstone, Edinburgh

Smith, V.N. and Bass, T.A. (1982) Problem solving techniques, *Communication for the Health Care Team*, Harper and Row, London, Ch. 9

Strongman, K.T. (1979) Attitudes and prejudices, *Psychology for the Paramedical Professions*, Croom Helm, London

CHAPTER 8

COUNSELLING

In Chapter 7 we explored the social problem solving process with specific reference to changing attitudes and prejudice through persuasion. A rather different application of a problem solving framework is discussed in this chapter as we consider counselling skills. Counselling may be seen to be a process whereby one person enables another constructively to resolve personal problem(s) that may be long standing or acute.

8.1 The counselling approach

There are times when the most helpful thing a nurse can do for someone else who has a problem is to provide the sort of conditions which will encourage that person to explore the problem and arrive at viable solutions her/himself. In these situations persuasion is no good, reassurance is difficult and advice giving is inappropriate. Take, for example, the case of a middle-aged man who has had surgery for a scrotal hernia. He appears worried that the pain he has is not controlled adequately:

P. I don't think I can cope with the pain but the doctor won't give me anything stronger. He says it'll stop hurting as soon as the wound heals, but I can't concentrate — even read the paper — because of it.

N. (*persuasion*) Just try to bear it a little longer: most men find they can.

or

(*sympathy*) I'm really sorry. It's always difficult coping with pain.

or

(*reassurance*) It does take time but I'm sure you'll soon begin to feel better.

or

(*information*) But it's not good for you to be on stronger drugs for this kind of problem — you might get constipated.

or

(*advice*) When you feel uncomfortable close your eyes and think of your favourite holiday spot. This will help.

None of these responses from the nurse will help the patient explore or understand the reasons for his pain and his reaction to it. Nor are they likely to produce lasting changes in the patient, as he had not taken an active part in reaching a solution. A very different effect would have been made had the nurse, for example, tried to encourage the patient to explore his concerns, as in, for example:

N. It seems as if the pain is making you frustrated. (*Encourages further disclosure through paraphrasing.*)

or

When do you feel the most pain? (*Encourages concreteness through the use of closed questions.*)

or

Is there anything about the operation and recovering from it that you feel you'd like to discuss further? (*Encourages exploration by moving the conversation on.*)

or

Does your wife know you're in a lot of pain? (*Moves conversation on by connecting with significant other.*)

These latter replies constitute part of what we call a counselling approach to helping. Nurses are often in situations that require them to develop a counselling relationship with another person or to use counselling skills in order to provide help and support for someone who is concerned or perplexed. Broadly, then, the main objectives of nurses as counsellors are:

(a) to create an atmosphere in which others feel accepted, understood and valued, so that they are helped to explore their thoughts, feelings and behaviour;

(b) to help others reach clearer understanding;
(c) to help others find their own strengths to cope more effectively with their lives by making appropriate decisions;
(d) to support and encourage alternative ways to act; and
(e) to help others evaluate the consequences of their actions, and to plan and engage in further actions if necessary.

This approach is what can be called an eclectic person-centred approach to counselling and is based on the works of Gerard Egan and Robert Carkhuff who in turn owe a lot to Carl Rogers. It is important to clarify this, so that we do not become confused with other approaches to counselling. Within this framework, two features distinguish counselling from other forms of helping. Firstly, if nurses are counselling, they are encouraging others to explore and understand their thoughts and feelings, and to work out what they might do *before* taking action. Secondly the role of the nurse is to help others form decisions or find solutions *of their own*. Counselling is not a better form of helping, it is a different one and is only the preferred form in some situations. Exercise 8.1 is designed to clarify those forms of helping that are most appropriate in different nursing situations.

Very often the transitory and emotionally charged nature of nurses' relationships with others, particularly patients, means that counselling relationships, extending over a period of time may be difficult to achieve. However, nurses may still be able to use some of the *skills* of counselling in order to enrich therapeutic personal relationships.

8.2 The counselling process

We have talked, above, of the counselling relationship and of counselling skills. It is the *relationship* that creates the helpful atmosphere in which the *skills* will be used to best effect, and in turn certain *skills* help create the helping *relationship*. So, for example, nurses who hope to be able to help others cope with their anxieties about forthcoming surgery will only be able to do so if they have skilfully developed a climate of warmth and trust. Counselling, then includes skills of building relationships and of helping: one cannot occur without the other.

A useful way to think about the skills involved in counselling is to look at different stages of the counselling process. A three-stage model of counselling is shown in Figure 8.1. Here, the counselling process leads the client to

Exercise 8.1   Counselling and other helping relationships

Instructions

1. Please give some examples of different kinds of helping activities that might be expected of nurses in the following categories.
2. When you have thought about the different kinds of helping relationships, try to construct a definition of *counselling* that distinguishes it from these other forms of helping.

Answer sheet

Giving advice:

Giving practical help:

Giving reassurance:

Giving information:

Giving sympathy:

Counselling:

Giving guidance:

Definition of counselling:

Please think about concerns brought by patients, relatives and colleagues, for which they need help. List them below and tick those for which counselling might be appropriate:

In the light of your answers, consider the discussion issues.

Discussion issues

1. Can counselling take place as part of a different kind of helping relationship?
2. What distinguishes counselling from other helping activities?
3. What barriers to effective counselling are there in nursing?
4. In which situations might colleagues benefit from counselling?
5. How easy would it be to counsel at work?

Comments

---

explore, understand and act, whilst the helping relationship seeks to establish warmth and rapport, to help clarify problem(s), to set goals and to realize certain courses of action and to evaluate their effectiveness.

Each stage requires counsellors to use specific sets of skills, with later stage(s) building on the skills of earlier stages, as shown in Table 8.1.

We would argue that all nurses need the skills facilitating exploration (Stage I), many nurses need the skills facilitating understanding (Stage II) and those nurses whose work brings them regularly into more formal counselling relationships need the skills facilitating action (Stage III). Many of the problems nurses have to help other people with are at the level of Stage I or II. For example, take the young woman who is confused about her reactions to her new baby:

The baby gets me down. I'm not saying I don't love her and I don't think people should have children and then go out and leave them. I know I'm really lucky, but ...

She may need help in clarifying and sorting out her conflicting feelings towards her baby and this may be an end in itself. Or take the middle-aged man who is overweight and has just suffered a heart attack:

I've always been lucky and I guess I always will. I might die — but then we all will one day. One thing, though, I'm not going to give up the good things: I like smoking too much.

He may need help in clarifying his feelings too, but may also need help in seeing what he is doing to himself and how his feelings affect other people (for example, his family) and what lines of action might be open to him. In other words, exploration can lead to understanding. There are many other examples of problems met by nurses which require them to use skills to facilitate exploration and understanding, and Exercise 8.2 offers the chance to consider some of them.

Figure 8.1   Three-stage model of the counselling process

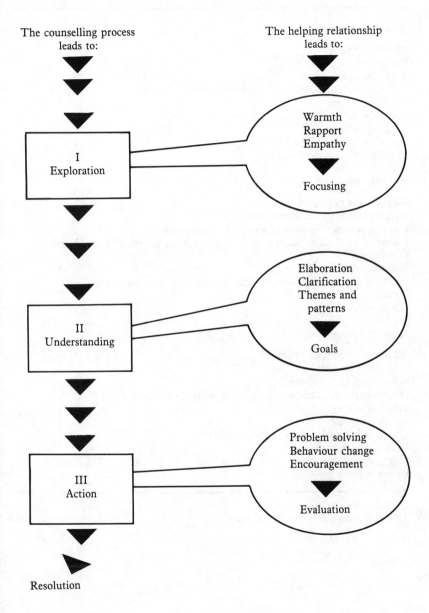

Table 8.1   Counselling skills for each stage of the counselling process

---

Stage I : Exploration

Attention-giving
Passive-listening
Active-listening
  Communicating empathy, acceptance, genuineness, by:
    Paraphrasing
    Reflecting thoughts and feelings
    Summarizing;
Focusing: helping client be specific
Moving conversations on

Stage II : Understanding

All the skills of Stage I
Helping the other clarify and elaborate ˙
Offering new perspectives or alternative frameworks
Listening for themes, patterns or gaps and helping the other recognize them
Comforting
Self-disclosure
Immediacy: what is happening between counsellor and the other, now
Timing
Goal-setting

Stage III : Action

All the skills of Stages I and II
Identifying strengths
Stimulating and encouraging
Divergent thinking and encouraging the other to be creative
Problem-solving
Decision-making
Changing behaviour and developing skills
Maintaining behaviour
Knowledge of resources
Evaluating

Exercise 8.2   Exploration: clarifying and understanding

Instructions

Please describe *three* situations you have met in your nursing practice where you think someone would have benefited from help in clarifying their problem(s). Describe each problem as fully as you can and given an indication of what that person might have gained from increased understanding.

Share your descriptions with a partner who has also completed the exercise, if possible, and discuss them in the light of the discussion issues.

Discussion issues

1. Is it ever enough to 'stop' at the exploration stage? Is understanding a reasonable goal in itself?
2. How do you know that understanding has been reached?
3. What factors inhibit nurses from encouraging patients to explore complex problems?

Comments

As understanding increases it can lead to decisions relating to how different strategies and lines of action might turn out. These can lead us to further explorations which in turn can lead to new insights and understanding and so on. Consider the young, active woman who suffered spinal injuries in a sporting accident and who has restricted mobility and a great deal of pain:

> I don't know how I'm going to manage — all the things I used to do I can't now. Where will I meet people? What can I do when I get so tired and the pain's so bad. Nothing helps.

Exploration, understanding and alternative courses of action are all indicated here, reflecting each stage of the counselling model.

We have seen then that nurses often have to use counselling skills in helping their patients, and those that are most frequently called for are those associated with Stages I and II of the counselling model. We will go on to consider these skills in some detail.

Skills facilitating exploration (stage I)

These skills are the most basic and indispensable of the counselling skills and can be used to good effect in many different nursing contexts. Table 8.1 gives a summary of the skills. Many of them have already been discussed as they overlap considerably within 'facilitation' skills (Chapter 5). Exercise 5.5 was an exercise in exploring listening skills. Effective use of questions (see Exercises 6.2 and 6.3) is essential for helpful listening. Listening in counselling is often an active process. It goes beyond attending to and receiving the message, and extends to communicating to the speaker that the facts and feelings have been heard and that the person is understood. *Paraphrasing, reflecting* thoughts and feelings and *summarizing* are all ways in which nurses can indicate that they understand, accept and empathize. Empathy is the ability to put ourselves in other people's shoes, to see a situation *as if* we were seeing it within their frames of reference. Non-verbal behaviour can indicate interest and attention (see Chapter 5), both necessary components of empathy. However, verbal skills are also required to convey our understanding to others. Exercise 8.3 offers the opportunity to explore the words we can use to express complex feelings.

We need a variety of words representing different feelings and *strengths* of feelings if we are to express our understanding accurately. Nurses meet people from different social groups and ethnic backgrounds, all of whom may have different colloquial expressions relating to bodily functions, medical procedures and emotional states. Exercise 8.3 also encourages exploration of colloquialisms. Paraphrasing and reflecting are two skills that help to communicate empathy. To paraphrase is to put what someone has said in different words without losing the essence of the original statement. Thus the use of synonyms and metaphors is required. Reflection is a form of paraphrasing that is generally limited to feelings. The purpose is to take all that another person says and to draw out the feelings contained therein both to show understanding and acceptance and to clarify them for that person.

Exercise 8.3   Descriptions of feelings

Instructions

1. Try to think of as many words for the different 'feeling states' and write them on the chart below. List all the words you can think of to represent different strengths of the feelings.

Feeling	Strong	Medium	Weak
Angry			
Happy			
Sad			
Afraid			
Disgusted			
Interested			
Confused			

2. Choose some feelings that you have experienced recently and write them in the present tense on the chart below (I feel perplexed, for example, I feel pleased, etc.). For each of these feelings, think of a colloquial expression that contains the feeling (for example, I'm like a chip waiting for its vinegar, I'm over the moon, etc.)

Feeling	Colloquial expressions

Discuss your answers with a partner who has also completed the exercise, if possible, in the light of the Discussion Issues.

Discussion issues

1. Are colloquial expressions understood by everyone? What does understanding depend on?
2. How might children refer to these feelings?

3. How would you refer to these feelings to your mother/grandmother/best friend?
4. Were any colloquialisms specific to geographical locations?
5. What implications does the lack of general understanding of colloquialisms have for nurses?

Comments

Consider the following strategies:

P. When I got the results I felt on top of the world — no more tests and samples.
N. I think you mean you were thrilled that the results mean no more investigations. (*Paraphrasing.*)
P. Yes, I was.
or
P. When I got the results I felt on top of the world — no more tests and samples.
N. It seems you were very pleased. (*Reflection.*)
P. Yes.

Note that in both these examples, the patient confirmed that the nurse had accurately picked up the feeling being expressed. Checking accuracy, and giving the other person the chance to clarify what she/he said, is important. In our example, the nurse uses statements to paraphrase and reflect instead of questions. This allows the other person to correct her/himself. The following exchange is an example of misunderstanding on the part of the nurse.

P. When I'm lying there day after day, I get to feel as if I'm falling further and further down a well, unable to climb out.
N. Despite your efforts, you feel very low, being in bed all day, then? (*Paraphrasing.*)
P. Yes and no. I certainly feel low, but I'm not making any effort. There's no point.
N. So everything seems hopeless. (*Reflection.*)
P. Yes.

In this example, the nurse uses a question instead of a statement to paraphrase, making it clear that she/he does not want to be corrected.

Paraphrasing and reflecting are, then, skills that are essential for Stage I of the counselling model and can be practised in Exercise 8.4. These skills may seem strange at first, but with practice they will become more natural.

To help others explore their problems, active listening (see Section 5.3) is vital. It is, however, sometimes not enough, and the skills of *focusing* and of *moving conversations on* have to be used, to encourage others to clarify their central concerns. Focusing may be used when people reveal complex concerns, with the different parts all mixed up, or when they make very general sweeping statements. Focusing helps them clarify and be more specific. For example, a young woman whose father is about to leave hospital following a stroke and will require home nursing:

Woman: I don't know how we'll cope with him at home. It'll be dreadful to see him so dependent, and I'm really so busy all day what with the children and one thing and another.

Nurse: It seems as if you have a lot of worries. What do you envisage to be the biggest problem for you? (*Focusing.*)

or

It seems as if it will be difficult for you. What is it that worries you most about your father being at home? (*Focusing.*)

or

We've talked about his dependence before. I wonder if we could consider for a moment how you will be able to organize your day as a family so you can manage? (*Moving the conversation on.*)

Focusing and moving conversations on are examined in Exercises 8.5 and 8.6, and methods of summarizing to move conversations on are shown in Table 8.2.

In this section we have briefly discussed some foundation counselling skills that help others explore their problems in order to bring about greater clarity. We will now go on to consider some of the skills that are required for Stage II of the counselling model (Figure 8.1), namely those skills that facilitate understanding.

Exercise 8.4   Paraphrasing and reflecting

Instructions

Paraphrasing

1. With a partner, allocate the roles A and B.
2. A — make a statement about yourself or about B.
3. B — reply to A with the words 'What I think you mean is ...' putting in your own words what you think A meant.
4. A — do not comment on B's statement.
5. A — make another statement which B is to paraphrase, starting with the words 'What I think you mean is ...'
6. Swop roles and repeat.
7. Discuss the experience with each other.
8. Repeat the exercise making statements about nursing as a profession. This time, after each paraphrase, tell your partner if she/he was right/wrong. If wrong, try another paraphrase until your partner finds it acceptable.
9. Discuss the experience.

Further paraphrasing

1. For each of the following statements, write down a list of the feeling(s) being expressed. Use simple words/phrases, and indicate the strength of feeling.

   (a) *26-year-old ward sister, newly appointed:* I need to build up my confidence for myself and be more assertive especially with the non-trained staff. They have an advantage over me — been here longer and think they know it all. And I suppose in one sense they do. But it can't be helped. They've got to do it my way. I don't really have the experience to draw on — but blow it! I'm well qualified and have done well. So we'll just have to see.
   She feels:

   (b) *Fifty-year-old man, on holiday from Australia, recovering from appendicectomy has just been informed by a policeman, accompanied by his sister in law, that his wife has been killed in a car accident. He is talking to staff nurse:* What do I do now? Do you think there might have been a mix-up? She's coming to see me after dinner. I can't believe it — it's *me* that's in hospital ... How can I take her home to bury her when I'm stuck in here? Do you think there'll be a postmortem?
   He feels:

(c) *Student nurse, discussing first day on ward with flat-mate:* I felt really chuffed in my uniform — thought it suited me and was just thinking 'I wish my Mum could see this', when I heard him calling 'nurse!' I didn't take any notice ... then I realized with horror it could only have been me he was calling. My heart missed a beat — what did he want? I couldn't let him know I was new. *She feels:*

(d) *Third-year student nurse talking to tutor:* The nerve of it! Who does he think he is? I was told by sister to join the ward round, and after the round he dragged me into the office and said what right had I to join *his* ward round without introducing myself and asking his permission. I was stunned into silence — it's not even as if he ever takes notice of us anyway! I'm livid — never been so humiliated in my life.
He feels:

2. In each case try to write down what the feeling was *about*. Summarize in as few words as possible, what circumstances or people are connected to the feelings.

   (a) The nurse's feelings are due to ...

   (b) The man's feelings are due to ...

   (c) The young woman's feeling are due to ...

   (d) The nurse's feelings are due to ...

3. Imagine each statement has been made to you. Try to reply to each 'person' by reflecting the feeling and relating it to the context you have identified. Be as concise but as accurate as you can.

   (a) Reply to nurse:
   It seems to me you feel...
   because...

   (b) Reply to man:
   It seems to me you feel...
   because...

   (c) Reply to friend:
   It seems to me you feel...
   because...

   (d) Reply to nurse:
   It seems to me you feel...
   because...

Reflecting

You have practised identifying the feeling and content areas of personal statements. This is now an opportunity to give this further practice and to receive feedback from someone else about your accuracy. With a partner, allocate roles A and B.

1. A — make a statement about yourself (take a topic from the list below if you like). Try to include some statement about feeling.
2. B — after each statement that A makes, try to paraphrase and reflect what has been said.
3. A — tell B whether or not she/he was accurate in her/his reflection.
4. Repeat for six statements from A.
5. Swop roles and repeat.
6. Discuss your experiences in this entire exercise with reference to the Discussion issues.

Topics for speakers

1. What I get the most satisfaction from at work ...
2. If I could change any aspect of myself as a nurse ...
3. What I hope to get out of nursing as a career is ...
4. I don't have time to do what I'd like to do, which is ...
5. What I feel about taking part in this course is ...
6. The most irritating patient in my experience is ...

Discussion issues

1. Did paraphrasing and reflecting become more 'accurate' as the exercise proceeded? Why/why not?
2. Is paraphrasing easier than reflecting? Why/why not?
3. What are the advantages of using statements rather than questions when reflecting (for example, 'What I think you mean is ...', 'I wonder if you feel ...', 'I think what you are saying is ...')
4. Are there some people with whom it would be difficult to paraphrase/reflect? Why?
5. Are there any situations where paraphrasing/reflecting might have adverse effects?
6. What does it feel like to be 'paraphrased/reflected'?

Comments

Table 8.2   Some methods of summarizing to move conversations on

---

At various stages during helping interview with another person it may be necessary to try to move the interview on. Summarizing can help to do this. Summarizing can also help end a lengthy interview and create a 'set' or expectation about the issues to be considered on a subsequent occasion.

Summarizing using a **contrast**

The summary includes a paraphrase of the issues and a suggestion that the speaker considers some alternatives that might be available.

E.g. You must have had a very unhappy time in hospital. I wonder, though, if you could look ahead and think how you'd feel if you just walked out, now, in the middle of your treatment.

Summarizing using a **choice point**

The summary includes a paraphrase of the issues and a suggestion that the speaker thinks about the various concerns and chooses one to work on.

E.g. You must have had a very unhappy time in hospital. There seem to be several things that are bothering you — not knowing what's wrong with you, worrying about dying so young as both your parents did and getting angry at the lack of consideration of the nursing staff. I guess we'll need to explore them all. Which do you think we should start on?

Summarizing using **figure-ground**, *i.e. identifying the uppermost issue*

The summary includes a paraphrase of the issues and a suggestion of which issue may be of the greatest concern.

E.g. You must have had a very unhappy time in hospital. There seem to be several things that are bothering you — not knowing what's wrong with you, worrying about dying so young and getting angry at the lack of consideration of the nursing staff. It feels as if your fear of dying is causing you most concern just now. I wonder if it would be useful to talk about that a bit more.

Exercise 8.5   Concreteness: general to specific

Instructions

1. Please write down three vague statements of recent experiences (for example, 'People have been nice to me'):

   (a)

   (b)

   (c)

2. Please give three concrete statements of experience (that is, what *actually* happened to you):

   (a)

   (b)

   (c)

3. Please write down three vague statements about behaviours (for example, 'I work inefficiently'):

   (a)

   (b)

   (c)

4. Please give three concrete statements about behaviour (that is, what did you *actually* do?):

   (a)

   (b)

   (c)

5. Please write down three vague statements of feelings that go with your experience and behaviour (for example, 'I'm happy to be with other people'; 'I get frustrated with the way I work'):

   (a)

   (b)

   (c)

6. Please give three concrete statements of feelings (that is, what did you *actually* feel and what did you feel like doing?)

(a)

(b)

(c)

7. Consider the discussion issues with a partner who has also completed the exercise if possible.

Discussion issues

1. How easy is it to be specific? Are some topics easier than others to be specific about? If so, why?
2. How comfortable would you feel asking a stranger to be more specific?
3. Can you think of an instance from your nursing experience where you have had to ask someone to be more specific? What was it like?
4. Are some types of question more helpful than others in encouraging concreteness? Why?
5. Would you use different types of question with people you know less well? Why?

Comments

Exercise 8.6 Summarizing to move conversations on

Instructions

With reference to Table 8.2, please consider the examples below. Construct suitable replies for each example. Your replies should include a summary of the issues and at least one of the following:
(a) a contrast; (b) a choice point; (c) a 'figure-ground'. You should try to devise a different means of moving on for each example.

Answer sheet

Case study

You are a student nurse on an antenatal ward. Elsie Jones wants to talk to you. She is expecting her second child in 6 weeks, and was admitted because of no weight gain. Her husband has left her for another woman with five children. She is now angry and frightened of coping with her new baby and 3-year-old alone. Her husband has offered to take their son for a while to help her out. (He does not want custody, but wants to reduce the strain on Elsie as far as possible.) The child wants to go. Elsie is confused and does not know what to do. She is also anxious about money and about how she will manage. She hopes her husband will come back.

Your reply to 'move her on':

Case study 2

You are a staff nurse on a general medical word. Mrs Lewis is an 84-year-old woman who was admitted 10 weeks ago following a fall in her third-storey flat, when she fractured her skull and her left arm. She has requested that the social worker makes sure she can return to her own flat. The social worker and ward staff all think that Mrs Lewis would be better living in local authority, warden-controlled housing. Mrs Lewis's granddaughter, who collects her pension every week and does her shopping for her, agrees. Mrs Lewis is in two minds whether or not to accept the proposition. She dearly wants her *own* flat, and is angry with her granddaughter, feeling she has betrayed her. She has come to rely on her granddaughter, but now says she is unable to do so. She is afraid she will die if she goes into sheltered accommodation.

Your reply to 'move her on':

Case study 3

You are a student nurse on a male orthopaedic ward. Adam is an active young man of 22 who broke both his legs and his right arm in a road accident in which a man died. His legs are not mending and he has had several bone grafts. His arm has healed but his writing is affected and is barely legible. He is worried that he will not be able to write acceptable job applications. Adam lost his job as a travelling salesman following his accident, and he feels bitter about this. He is despondent that he lacks any skills that might get him a job although he is considering a government training course. He refuses to attend occupational therapy and sits smoking in the day room all day, 'festering' as he calls it. He is convinced that the accident was his fault although the inquest returned a verdict of accidental death. He lacks confidence that he will ever work again or that women will find him attractive if he limps.

Your reply to 'move him on':

In the light of the replies you have constructed, consider the discussion issues.

Discussion issues

1. Were any forms of summary easier to devise than others? Why?
2. Which form of summary would be the most effective? Why?
3. Can you think of examples from your nursing practice where these summaries were/would be appropriate?

Comments

Skills facilitating understanding (stage II)

The skills that facilitate understanding help people who have problems see things more objectively and from new perspectives, as well as help them increase their self-awareness and set themselves (appropriate) goals (see Table 8.1). We have considered some of these skills earlier (for example, self-disclosure, Exercise 5.7), and all those discussed above are relevant too. In Stage II of the counselling model, people with problems are challenged so that they develop greater understanding of their problems and acceptable goals to be aiming for. Consider the case of the colleague who cannot decide whether to apply for a job:

Colleague: I can't decide what to do. I think I should try for it but I'm not sure I'd even get an interview. That would be terrible. I'd feel awful ...
Nurse: You've mentioned how bad 'failure' in applying for jobs would be for you before. It seems as if this is an issue for you. (*Identification of theme.*)
Colleague: Oh, I don't think so — no. (*Evasion.*)
Nurse: It seems as if it is. You will need to face up to this if you are seriously thinking of your career. (*Challenge.*)

Colleague: Hm. Perhaps you're right ...

Nurse: What is it that concerns you about failure in interviews? (*Focusing.*)

Colleague: Well, everyone should be successful shouldn't they?

Nurse: Why 'should'? (*Challenge.*)

Colleage: That's obvious — everyone wants success.

Nurse: Not necessarily — there may be other reasons people stay on or move out of jobs. (*Offers alternative perspective.*)

or

Colleague: I can't decide what to do: I think I should try for it but I'm not sure I'd even get an interview. That would be terrible. I'd feel awful.

Nurse: What makes you think you wouldn't get an interview? (*Focusing.*)

Colleague: Oh I'm not nearly good enough. I've nothing to offer.

Nurse: But you're well liked, good at making decisions and keep your head in a panic. (*Identifying strengths.*)

These techniques usually emerge in the course of a helping relationship, and, as a rule, they should not be used in the exploratory stage, where non-directive skills are of more value. It is worth practising some of these skills, as nurses frequently do develop helping relationships that extend over a period of time. Exercise 8.7 highlights the identification of strengths. The overall aim of helping people understand their problem(s) is to enable them to set themselves realistic goals that they can go on to achieve. To be realistic, goals should be concrete or specific rather than vague; clear and easy to establish when they have been reached; within a person's scope and capabilities; within a person's values; and attainable over a reasonable period of time. Practice at setting realistic goals is offered in Exercise 8.8.

Having reached the stage of better understanding and the setting of goals, the issue remains of how to act so that the goals can be met. This brings us to the helping skills that facilitate action.

Skills facilitating action (stage III)

We have suggested, above, that nurses have perhaps less need of these skills than of those facilitating exploration and understanding. We have examined the social problem solving process elsewhere (see Chapter 7, Exercises 7.1 and 7.2) but it is also relevant here. Some Stage III skills are too specialized to be included here (such as those of behaviour change and maintenance). However, we think that some of the techniques that encourage divergent thinking and that help reflect on barriers to change are useful.

Exercise 8.7   Identification of personal strengths

Instructions

This exercise is best done with a partner.

Working by yourself, write a list of your own strengths as (a) a friend, and (b) a nurse. Share your list with your partner. Tell your partner what you think her/his strengths are. Listen to what your partner tells you: summarize what you have heard, starting with the words 'It seems as if you think I ...'. Swop roles and repeat.

Take it in turns to talk about one strength you think your partner has, but does not use enough (try not to discuss the accuracy of the judgements). Discuss the experience of doing the exercise with reference to the discussion issues.

Discussion Issues

1. What barriers prevent you using your strengths to best effect (think of examples from work if possible).
2. Could you have told someone you did not know well what you thought her/his strengths were? Why/why not?
3. Could you have told your parents/other close relatives what you thought their strengths were? Why/why not?
4. Does nursing encourage you to examine your strengths?

Comments

Exercise 8.8   Setting realistic goals

Instructions

1. Please identify two general aims you have. Consider how these aims can be made more specific until they have evolved into specific goals for action.

Example

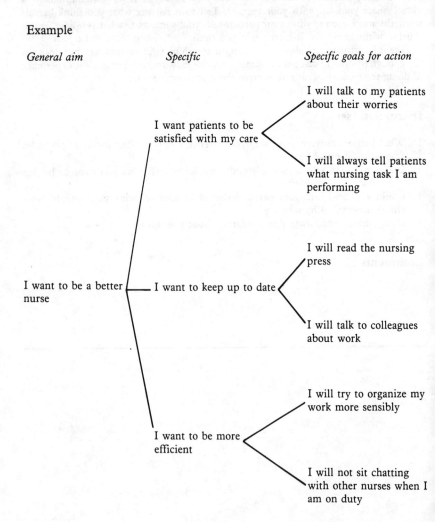

General aim	*Specific*	*Specific goals for action*
I want to be a better nurse	I want patients to be satisfied with my care	I will talk to my patients about their worries
		I will always tell patients what nursing task I am performing
	I want to keep up to date	I will read the nursing press
		I will talk to colleagues about work
	I want to be more efficient	I will try to organize my work more sensibly
		I will not sit chatting with other nurses when I am on duty

Answer sheet

General aim   *Specific aim*   *Specific goals for action*

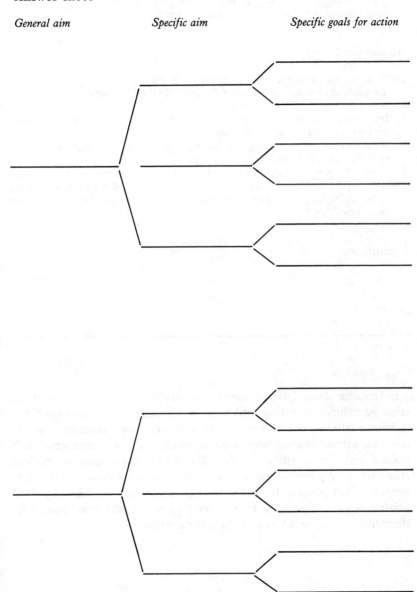

2. With a partner, if possible one has also completed the exercise, please consider your answers in the light of the discussion issues.

Discussion issues

1. What are the advantages of setting realistic goals?
2. Are goals more easily set in some spheres of life than in others? Why might this be?
3. Have you ever been in a position, at work, to help someone else set realistic goals for themselves? If so, please describe.
4. What barriers are there in nursing that might prevent or encourage the setting of realistic goals for (a) patients and (b) nurses?
5. What strategies do you use to prevent patients setting themselves realistic goals with respect to their capabilities in the context of their illnesses? (Examine the verbal strategies you frequently use, such as 'jollying them along', 'keeping up their hopes', etc.)

Comments

In thinking about different ways that a person may act for change, it can often be helpful to 'brainstorm' ideas or possibilities. Brainstorming is a technique whereby one or more people think of as many associated ideas as they can, without rejecting any. Some of the ideas will be conventional, some unusual and some wildly impossible. Brainstorming is a means of thinking creatively about a problem, and to arrive at ideas for solutions that might be unusual — but possible. It is a way to help people think more broadly about possible courses of action at times when they would otherwise be stuck for alternatives. Exercise 8.9 is a brainstorming session.

Exercise 8.9   Brainstorming

Instructions

This exercise is best carried out in small groups (of up to 6 people) although it is possible to do it individually or in pairs.
1. Take one of the problems listed below. Consider as many possible courses of action in response to the problem as you can, and write them down. Include everything that comes to mind; do not reject any idea, however bizarre or impossible it seems.
2. After about 5 minutes of 'brainstorming', discuss the most viable and the least viable solutions, with reasons for the choices.
3. Repeat the procedure for each of the problems below.
4. When you have agreed a set of viable solutions for all the problems, consider the discussion issues.

Problems

1. Mother, whose diabetic 8-year-old child will not stick to her diet.
2. Teenage lad on orthopaedic ward who refuses to have long hair treated for head lice.
3. Five-year-old boy with a squint who cannot be relied upon to keep occlusive eye patch in place.
4. Forty-year-old fashion model who cannot look at her mastectomy wound four weeks after surgery.
5. Incontinent elderly woman who forgets to tell staff that she needs to go to the toilet.

Discussion issues

1. How easy is brainstorming?
2. How does the number of people discussing the problem effect the number or quality of ideas produced?
3. What might inhibit your attempts to 'brainstorm' with patients? (e.g. role, personal inhibitions, lack of knowledge, etc.)
4. Do cultural differences affect brainstorming? How?

Comments

Let us take, for example, the 35-year-old man with psoriasis, who leads a hectic life. He easily forgets to take his medication with any regularity, with consequent episodes with florid symptoms. Brainstorming around the question 'How can I remember to take my medication' may lead to solutions such as rehearsing a schedule every morning; writing a memory note in his diary every day; pinning notices up in his office at work; buying a watch with hourly alarm settings; asking a colleague to telephone him when his pill is due; putting the light on a time switch to come on at the time his pill is due; arranging his pill schedule to coincide with other regular events (such as tea/coffee times, dinner, etc.), and so on. Some solutions may be viable, and may work!

When we help others consider and take various actions for themselves, it can help to examine, with them, some of the possible barriers that might impede their progress. It can be useful to do this before they actually take any measures, so they can be realistic in their expectations for success or not. Take, for example, the case of an elderly woman with terminal cancer who has been living with her daughter but now thinks she wants to return to her own home 'to die'. The district nurse has been helping her explore her concerns and to arrive at a definite solution. They have explored the issues and the woman has decided her goal *is* to go home. What are the pressures or forces that might impede a successful return? We can consider the problem in terms of a 'force-field' analysis. As we can see from Figure 8.2 a force-field analysis requires us to identify those forces that hinder progress towards a goal and those that facilitate progress. Then the task is to help another person decrease hindering forces and increase and strengthen facilitating forces. So, in our example it may be that there are many restraining forces such as daughter's objections, woman's inability to care adequately for herself, district nurses' case loads, age, and so on. These will hinder her chances of a successful return

Figure 8.2   Force-field analysis

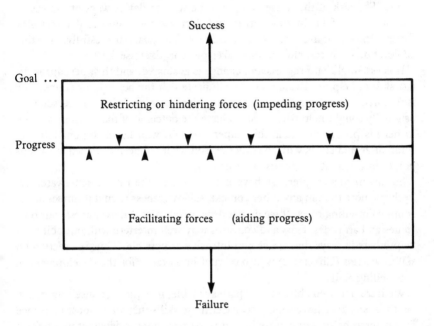

Personal forces

Disposition (e.g.)
  optimistic
  caring
  selfish
  thoughtful
  imaginative
  impatient
Age
Health
Skills

Situational forces

Family
Friends
Job
Locality
Finances
Commitments
Mobility
Housing
Services

home. However there may also be facilitating forces such as her commitment, friends' support, district nurse's support, proximity of shops to her home, and so on. The task of the nurse is to help the woman devise ways of increasing the numbers of facilitating forces and decrease the number of restraining forces, thus helping the woman achieve her goal successfully. Further exploration of force-field analyses takes place in Exercise 8.10.

It is essential that progress and change is evaluated, and this, perhaps is the last skill of helping. Evaluation may indicate that further help or counselling is required or it may indicate that the problem is 'solved'. It is the person who originally sought help who must evaluate the outcome of that help in relation to her/his problem(s). It is the helper, though, who has a responsibility to summarize and check with the other person what has been achieved at various points throughout the counselling process.

So far, in this chapter, we have not considered the role of self-awareness. Perhaps more than in any other context, self-awareness is vital if nurses are to adopt counselling roles. If we do not develop our own self-awareness, our own values and attitudes, fears and concerns may well interfere with our ability to help others in ways that are as non-intrusive as possible. Thus the section on self-awareness (Chapter 2) is also of vital importance for the development of counselling skills.

We have not been able, in the space available, to explore counselling in any depth. Instead we have sought to select those skills that are of most relevance for nurses as helpers or counsellors. It is, perhaps appropriate that we end this chapter by looking at constraints that may affect the successful resolution of personal problems. In Chapter 9 we are going to consider constraints that may affect the successful deployment of interpersonal skills by nurses.

Exercise 8.10 Force-field analysis

Instructions

This exercise is best carried out with a partner, but you can do it on your own if necessary.

Please look carefully at the example of a force-field analysis given below. Take about 10 minutes to discuss it. Now think of a problem you have had at work. With your partner, together work out a force-field analysis of the problem. Consider ways of reducing the restraining forces and of increasing the facilitating forces. Try to think about the balance between the forces at the moment. When you have each thought of a problem and done force-field analyses on them, consider the discussion issues.

Example of force-field analysis

A 48-year-old ward sister has been working on an orthopaedic ward for the past 15 years. She is competent, well regarded and confident that she does her work well. For the past three years she has developed a strong interest in moving into nurse education, although she has not studied for some time and is unsure of her academic ability. The school of nursing is considerably further from her home than the hospital and she does not drive. She wants regular weekends off duty because she and her husband have just bought a caravan in the Lake District. Her interest in moving into education was prompted by one of the senior tutors, who was keen to have her join the team because of the interest and skill she had shown in teaching students over the years. The Director of Nursing Services wants her to stay in the clinical field and has suggested that there may be a nursing officer post vacant on her unit, for which she will be encouraged to apply.

Steps in a force-field analysis

1. Identify the restraining forces.

2. Identify the facilitating forces.

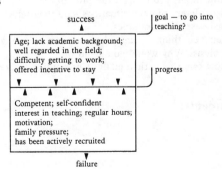

3. Decide on the balance of restraining/facilitating forces and represent this with arrows pointing in opposite directions.
4. Insert the 'progress' line in an appropriate place, taking into account the balance of restraining and facilitating forces.

Answer sheet

Force-field analysis of problem at work

Problem:

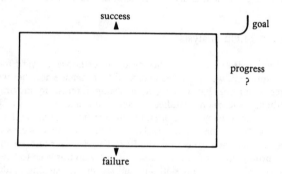

Discussion issues

1. What problems were there in doing the force-field analysis?
2. What might inhibit nurses from conducting force-field analyses with patients? How might you explain the procedure?
3. Do different nursing situations lend themselves more readily to using force-field analyses? Give examples.
4. Can you think of any circumstances where you would *not* use a force-field analysis? Why would you avoid it?
5. How can a force-field analysis be applied if there is no clear goal?

Comments:

8.3 Summary

This chapter has been concerned with some of the essential components of counselling skills. Specifically, the following points were raised:

Counselling is a form of helping wherein one person enables another to engage in constructive resolution of personal problems.

Counselling is a special form of helping and different in kind from persuasion, reassurance, advice, guidance and sympathy.

Counselling enables other people to find solutions of their own after fully exploring their thoughts, feelings and behaviours.

A person-centred approach to counselling seeks to create a trusting atmosphere in which others feel accepted, understood and valued.

Counselling aims to help others to reach clearer understanding and to find their own strengths in order to make appropriate decisions.

Counsellors support and encourage alternative ways to act and help others evaluate the consequences of their actions.

Nurses are able to make use of counselling skills even if they rarely develop long-term counselling relationships.

A warm, trusting atmosphere is a prerequisite of helping.

The counselling process can be viewed in terms of three stages: exploration, understanding and action.

Specific skills relate to different stages of the counselling process, although later stages incorporate skills of earlier ones.

Many nurses can make good use of skills facilitating exploration and understanding and fewer can use those facilitating action.

Skills relating to different stages of the counselling process may be used concurrently.

Skills facilitating exploration help develop a warm relationship, communicate empathy and help the other person focus on specific issues.

Skills facilitating understanding help people who have problems see things more objectively and from new perspectives as well as enabling them to set realistic goals for themselves.

Skills facilitating action help people plan and carry out suitable courses of action in order to attain their goals.

Force-field analysis is a problem solving method that examines the restraints on movement towards specified goals so that they can be decreased.

Evaluation and checking are essential throughout the counselling process.

Self-awareness in the counsellor is vital for effective helping.

Further reading

Egan, G. (1981) *The Skilled Helper* (2nd edn), Brooks Cole, Monterey
French, P. (1983) Counselling skills, *Social Skills for Nursing Practice*, Croom Helm, London, ch. 6
Nurse, G. (1981) *Counselling and the Nurse* (2nd edn), H.M. and M. Aylesbury
Oldfield, S. (1983) *The Counselling Relationship*, Routledge and Kegan Paul, London
Stewart, W. (1983) *Counselling in Nursing: a problem solving approach*, Harper and Row, London
Tschudin, V. (1982) *Counselling Skills for Nurses*, Baillière Tindall, London

CHAPTER 9

CONSTRAINTS ON USING EFFECTIVE INTERPERSONAL SKILLS

The effective use of interpersonal skills depends to a large extent on the context in which they are deployed. However interpersonally skilled we are we may find that our relationships are constrained by factors outside our control. A nurse who is trying to talk to a deaf patient in a noisy crowded room in an understaffed facility where the onus is on physical rather than patient-centred care may well find that her/his efforts are in vain. In this example, the nurse is coming up against factors relating to the patient (deafness), the physical setting (noise, crowding), priorities and funding of health care (understaffing), the organization (physical care emphasis) and possibly her/himself (frustration). In order to try to overcome some of these factors, the nurse must, first of all, learn to recognize them. Even then, though, there will be some factors (such as policy relating to health funding) that she/he will not be able to do anything about. Nurses' recognition of these factors though may help them evaluate their own interpersonal skills realistically. The questions we should ask are: *To what extent do features of the context put realistic constraints on my ability to use interpersonal skills effectively?* and *To what extent can I adjust my own interpersonal skills in order to make them more effective?*

In this chapter we will look at the context of nursing and explore the range of constraints that surrounded nurses' use of interpersonal skills, as shown in Figure 9.1.

Figure 9.1   Constraints on the effective use of interpersonal skill

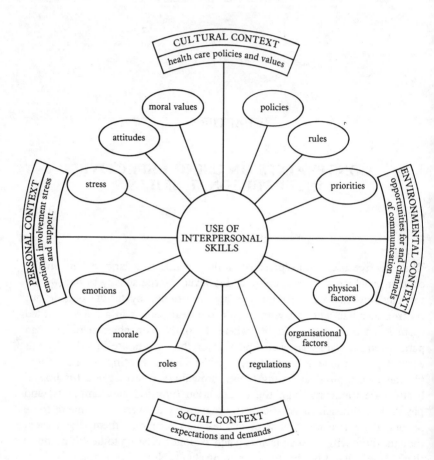

We will examine the personal, social and environmental features as well as some of the wider cultural aspects of nursing, with a view to gaining some insight into the extent to which we can deploy effective interpersonal skills as nurses.

9.1 Personal constraints

Until fairly recently, nurses were not expected to 'get involved' with their patients. It was considered 'professional' to remain detached and any personal involvement was a breach of professional etiquette. With an emphasis on the interpersonal aspects of nursing, this situation is changing. Nurses are now expected to 'get involved' with their patients in order to best assess their needs, and plan and deliver total patient care. This change of emphasis puts enormous pressure on nurses, and the role of the 'self' and self-awareness is central. We have explored some aspects of self-awareness in Chapter 2, and it may be useful here, to repeat some of these exercises with a particular interest in the effect of 'self' on the use of interpersonal skills.

Although nurses are expected to get involved with patients they are not expected to experience the range of emotions that they might experience in other relationships. They are not expected to feel angry, hurt, guilty, hostile, afraid, loving, and so on. And yet, of course, they do. We saw in Exercise 2.7 that if we feel unable to gain some control over events we are in danger of experiencing stress. Too much stress can lead to illness (physical and psychological — indigestion, headaches, depression/anxiety), low morale and lack of job satisfaction, all of which, in turn, can lead to nurses giving up their jobs in favour of an occupation that doesn't exact such a high personal price.

Development of relationships

The implementation of the nursing process and the adoption of an interpersonal approach to nursing both put pressures on the individual nurse to form good, warm and often therapeutic relationships with patients. This is, in itself, a strange thing to do. In the course of our everyday lives we form relationships out of choice and over a long period of time. Exercise 9.1 offers the opportunity to look at the way relationships with patients develop compared with those of good friends and professional colleagues.

Exercise 9.1   Development of relationships

Instructions

Please think of (a) a close friend, (b) a work colleague, and (c) a patient you have been nursing a lot recently. Think about your relationships with these people, and complete the questionnaire below.

Answer sheet

	Close friend	Work colleague	Patient
1. Did you have any choice whether or not you first spoke to this person?			
2. Did this person have any choice whether or not she/he spoke to or got to know you?			
3. How long did it take for this person to talk about her/his worries or concerns?			
4. Did you ever talk about your worries or concerns to this person?			
5. Do you share any interests?			
6. Have you touched this person? (a) clothed? (b) unclothed?			
7. How long had you known this person before you touched her/him?			
8. Has this person touched you? (a) clothed? (b) unclothed?			
9. Have you spoken to this person in the night?			
10. Have you been with this person (a) at bed time? (How long had you known her/him?) (b) at bath time? (How long had you known her/him?) (c) on a Sunday? (How long had you known her/him?) (d) for breakfast? (How long had you known her/him?)			

11. In how many different situations have you been with this person?
12. Has this person met any of your friends? How many?
13. If you found that you did not like this person, would you be able to break off your relationship?
14. If you were not going to see this person again, would you be able to say goodbye?
15. Can you make arrangements to see this person whenever you want?
16. Can this person make arrangements to see you whenever she/he wants?
17. Have you ever got angry with this person?
18. Have you ever cried in front of this person?
19. Has this person ever cried in front of you?
20. Have you ever shared experiences with this person that made you both laugh uncontrollably?

Consider your answers to the questions in the light of the discussion issues.

Discussion issues

1. How similar are relationships with patients to other personal relationships?
2. How similar are relationships with patients to other professional relationships?
3. Are relationships with patients two-way? In what ways?
4. Does the particular nursing setting influence the way you develop relationships with patients? How?
5. Does the age/sex/nationality of the patients affect the way you develop relationships with them? How?

Comments

It is likely that the replies in Exercise 9.1 reveal a picture of relationships with patients developing in part as those with colleagues do, and in part as those with good friends. Thus relationships with patients do not fit easily into a pattern with which we are familiar with in other walks of life. They are distinct and different. Nurses are expected to do intimate, personal things to patients, to share intimate, personal activities with them and to discuss intimate, personal issues with them but at the same time to reveal little that is intimate or personal about themselves. Most relationships, elsewhere, have an element of reciprocity (sharing) in them. Of course it can be argued that nurses have *role* relationships and not *personal* relationships with patients and it is this that distinguishes them (we will consider some of the implications of this later in the chapter [see Section 9.2]). Nevertheless, nurses do get embroiled in the intimate, personal lives of their patients, and the consequent drain on their emotional energy may have direct repercussions for patient care.

In addition to this, the very existence of particular emotional states (hostility, fear, anger, frustration, etc.) can distort the use of interpersonal skills at all levels (what is said, how it is said, how things are perceived, what courses of action are decided upon, etc.).

Personal support systems

One way in which the stressful effects of the emotional involvement nurses experience can be reduced is by setting up personal support systems. For some people, personal support is built into the job. Many psychiatric nurses for example have frequent case conferences or 'supervision' sessions, in which they can vent their feelings about their work, themselves and the people in their care. For others, interpersonal networks are built up, wherein groups of nurses often discuss their work and their involvement in it. Others, though, have no opportunity to air their feelings. Family and friends do not like them continually 'talking shop', and colleagues all seem to give the appearance of 'coping'. These are the nurses who are liable to experience the unpleasant effects of stress. Exercise 9.2 attempts to clarify those features of support systems that would go some way to reducing the stress on nurses.

Nursing will always involve a high emotional commitment. However, there is no reason why nurses' emotions should necessarily intrude upon their everyday activities and distort their interpersonal skills. Self-awareness is the first step to being able to overcome the constraints that emotions and personal

Exercise 9.2   Professional support systems

Instructions

In groups of six or individually, please think about how you would form a professional support group to meet your emotional and professional needs at work. Use the following questions as guidelines and prepare a case that could be put to the Director of Nursing Services for the introduction of professional support groups. Write your 'case' in not more than 250 words.

Guidelines

Necessity for support group

1. What situations arouse emotions in you, as a nurse, at work?
2. What opportunities do you have to discuss work with colleagues?
3. Which colleagues do you spend most time talking to about work?
4. How immediate are chances to talk about events at the time of stress?
5. Can you talk to anyone at work about serious personal problems?

Establishing a support group

1. What should members have in common (expertise, interest, etc.)?
2. What size should the group be?
3. Where/when should the group meet?
4. How similar/dissimilar should the members be?
5. Should members of the other health professions be included?
6. To what extent should relationships within the group be reciprocal?
7. Should attendance at the group be compulsory?
8. How confidential should the working of the group be?
9. Who will lead the group?

Expectations of the support group

1. To what extent should the group give members the opportunity to complain about their work/colleagues etc.?
2. Will the group offer people psychotherapy?
3. How comfortable will members feel during/after meetings?
4. How will stress be alleviated by membership of the support group?

Further issues

Share your 'case' with others who have also done the exercise, if possible, and consider the discussion issues.

Discussion issues

1. What barriers to setting up support groups at work might there be?
2. Why have nurses failed to establish support groups in the past?
3. Are formal support systems any advantage over informal ones?

Comments

---

involvement place on effective interpersonal skills use, and the building of appropriate support systems is the next one. Ideally, we should reach a stage where nurses are able to use 'self' in a therapeutic way, but this will require time and practice in self-exploration and an acknowledgement from the nursing profession at all levels that nurses need and must have personal support at work.

9.2 Social constraints

Social aspects of the nursing context refer in part to the actual people involved in a particular nursing activity. It makes no sense to talk of nurses' interpersonal skills in isolation from other people. Nurses have interaction partners, be these patients, colleagues, other health workers, relatives, etc. and they all constitute the *interaction context*.

Roles

All these people have roles and associated responsibilities: we have explored the concept of role and its implications for interpersonal skills in Chapter 4.

When different people are present in a nursing setting, though, the situation itself may be re-defined and this in turn will dictate or prohibit particular repertoires of interpersonal skill. In a hospital ward, for example, different people enter at different times during the day, radically changing the situation for everyone concerned, affecting both the way it is perceived and the behaviours that are expected. When the consultant's team enters the ward, nurses (and patients) act differently from when the visitors arrive. It is not the people themselves that have made the difference but the understanding of the roles they occupy.

We have seen above that nurses might behave differently *in* their role of nurse than out of it. Patients, too, may behave in unpredictable ways that bear little resemblance to their general social behaviour outside the patient role. Patients are ill. Their illnesses may be distressing, painful, distorting of senses such as sight, hearing, touch or even consciousness. Thus patients, too, might experience increased emotion and distress, which may in turn, distort their interactions. It is sometimes suggested that patients are encouraged by health personnel to conform to the 'good' sick role. They are allowed to abdicate their normal social responsibilities and are exempted from responsibility for their conditions, but at the same time are expected to cooperate in order to get well. The 'bad' patients are the uncooperative, questioning people who appear to lack the will to get better. Generally nurses dislike grumbling, complaining, questioning and demanding patients, and liking affects the use of interpersonal skills. It is often argued that it is the ability to overcome factors such as this that distinguish the interpersonal skills of the professional from the lay person. Exercise 9.3 is designed to explore the ways liking/disliking constrains interpersonal skills in nursing.

It may be useful to look again at Exercise 4.1 which focuses on the demands and expectations brought to bear on the role of the nurse. Other social factors that may affect interactions include whether or not all the people in a particular situation are of the same age, sex, ethnic background, and so on. The relative importance of these factors is difficult to predict and will relate to everyone's past experience, stereotypes and prejudices (see Section 7.2).

Regulations

In most nursing contexts there are regulations that tell people who occupy different roles how to behave or what to do. These regulations may be clearly stated (explicit) or assumed (implicit). We have considered social rules

Exercise 9.3   The influence of liking and disliking on interpersonal skills

---

Instructions

Please think of a patient you (a) like and one you (b) dislike. Consider briefly what it is you like/dislike about them. Try to list as many ways you think your interpersonal behaviour is influenced by your feelings towards (a) and (b).

Example

(a) Smiles, co-operates, says nice things to me.

I stop to talk whenever I can. Talk about myself. Try to be the one to accompany her to the bathroom. Take time to really listen to her concern and to answer any questions she has. etc. etc.

(b) Shouts, sulks, tries to get attention all the time.

Avoid. Don't look at her when I have to talk to her. Give excuses for leaving her (not true!) Snap at her when she's going on. Make her feel guilty about effect on other patients. Give no opportunity for her to express her worries. Say I don't know too easily etc. etc.

Answer sheet

(a)   (b)

Share your answers with a partner and identify similarities in how you deal with the two people. Consider the discussion issues.

Discussion issues:

1. To what extent do nurses 'overcompensate' when they know they dislike patients? What effect does this have?
2. To what extent does the way nurses relate to irritating patients encourage them in their irritating ways? How?
3. What happens to patients that are neither strongly liked or disliked?
4. What happens if *patients* like or dislike particular nurses?
5. Are particular 'types' of patients more likely to be liked/disliked (e.g. age, culture, disorder, sex, class, etc.) and in what ways?

Comments

---

elsewhere (Chapter 4) but it is useful to think further of how the regulations may constrain the effective deployment of interpersonal skills by nurses. For example, a regulation that there must be two trained nurses administering a drug round might mean that neither of them can have a conversation with a distressed patient whilst the round is in progress. A regulation that patients may only smoke in the day room may mean that a nurse who finds a smoky atmosphere extremely unpleasant may avoid the day room and thereby miss the opportunity to talk in a relaxed atmosphere with patients (or she/he may be so irritated by having to talk in the smoky room that the quality of the interaction is affected. The smoke may similarly affect non-smoking patients). The regulation that parents may not eat on a children's ward may result in unnecessary confrontations between nurses and parents as the nurses try to enforce the regulations. The regulation that visitors must wait for the screens to be drawn back before entering the ward may mean that a crowd of angry relatives and friends may come into the ward if there has been some delay. There are many other examples of how regulations can constrain the use of interpersonal skills (see Exercise 9.4). Regulations of the sort mentioned above are closely tied to the organizational context of nursing.

Organizational factors

Organizational factors are those that relate to the ways that nursing activities are structured, and these can constrain nurses' freedom to use their interpersonal skills as they would like to. In hospitals, the ways in which wards are organized may curtail the opportunities for talking with patients. For example, nurses may spend a great deal of time filling in the Kardex system, or on the phone to other departments. In the community, too, the

Exercise 9.4   Regulations

Instructions

In the most recent nursing setting that you worked in, think about the ways in which regulations constrained the use of interpersonal skills. Try to make sure you think about explicit/implicit regulations; setting — specific/professional regulations; those that affect the opportunities for interaction/quality of interaction and so on.

Discuss your answers with a partner and discuss further examples if you can.

Answer sheet

Regulations

Effect on interpersonal skill use

E.g. As soon as the phone in the office rings it must be answered.

E.g. Prematurely cuts off personal conversations with patients.

Discussion issues

1. Do any regulations encourage the use of interpersonal skills?
2. What happens when a patient/relative/staff member is not aware of the regulations?
3. On what basis might you decide to break a regulation?
4. Are there some regulations that should never be broken? What?
5. What do you do if you find someone breaking a regulation?
6. What happens when a patient refuses to acknowledge the need for a particular regulation?

Comments

requirements of administration, the writing of letters, making phone calls and so on, may take up considerable time. These tasks may also contribute to nurses' frustration, and have consequences for mood and thereby interactions (if say the number of phones is restricted, or calls can only be made after one o'clock, etc.). Shift work may mean that once good relationships are formed, they cannot be pursued and partings may not be possible. Patients therefore may experience several beginnings to relationships over two/three days and nurses may not see any relationships through over the same period. Thus both are relating in unpredictable circumstances and may well feel frustrated as a result. Exercise 9.5 attempts to identify the ways different organizational factors affect the use of interpersonal skills.

Many of the organizational aspects of the nursing context are identified in Exercise 9.5 and will contribute to what we can call the *organizational climate*. The organizational climate affects the well-being of the people working within it, and this in turn affects their interpersonal behaviour. Several things influence the quality of the organizational climate. For example, the amount of autonomy people are given, coupled with the degree of consideration, warmth and support they receive from their superiors will affect morale. If nurses are allowed no autonomy, or are given too much too soon, they may develop a lack of self-confidence or anxiety at the responsibility they are expected to bear. If their work is highly structured and supervised too stringently, again they might develop a lack of confidence which results in a reluctance to take decisions in conversations with patients. There are several interesting things about the effect of organizational climate on people at work. The climate is a *perceived* one and not everyone will react in the same way to the same organizational context. Furthermore, people at different stages of their careers may respond differently to particular organizational practices. So, it may well be that student nurses *gain* confidence from highly structured and supervised work settings but more senior nurses do *not*. Thus the organizational climate will have different affects on different people's skills.

We have noted above, that organizational factors can not only put constraints on the opportunities for interaction, but also affect the level of morale of nurses at work. The environmental context, too, can put similar constraints on the use of interpersonal skill.

Exercise 9.5 Organizational constraints on the use of interpersonal skills

---

Instructions

Please think about the ways that organizational factors may affect the use of interpersonal skills by nurses. Try to think about direct and indirect consequences of organizational aspects of your work.

Discuss your answers with a partner and generate further examples if you can.

Answer sheet

Organizational factor	*Effect on interpersonal skills use*
Examples:	Examples:
Phones do not have outside lines	Less time to talk with patients
Night staff 'do' breakfasts	Patients are unnecessarily tired and
Lack of coordination between	therefore snappy
departments	Frustration (indirect)
No opportunity to make decisions	Evasion when asked direct questions
	Defer to another authority etc.

With a partner, if possible one who has also completed the exercise, consider the discussion issues.

Discussion issues

1. Can you identify any organizational factors that make it easier to use effective interpersonal skills.
2. How does the bureaucracy of the health services affect nurses' use of interpersonal skills?
3. Do organizational factors affect relationships with colleagues/relatives/patients most? In what ways?
4. How can changes to organization be made so as to remove the constraints on nurses' use of interpersonal skills? (This could be the topic for a good brainstorming session: see Exercise 8.9)

Comments

9.3 Environmental constraints

By environmental constraints we are referring to the physical aspects of nursing contexts and the associated rules for acting within them.

Physical environment

The physical layout of a nursing setting will encourage certain interactions and discourage others. It has been shown time and time again that if we pass others often, we are likely to talk to them. So, patients near the nursing office, near the doorways of the wards, near the dayroom, etc. are more likely to be talked to than those more distant from the amenities or the 'routes' of activity. Highly polished floors may prevent patients who are a little unsteady on their feet finding a nurse in order to initiate conversation. (Highly polished floors or long corridors with nowhere to rest encourage patients to stay in an inactive sick role!) Nurses who spend a lot of time in the office or kitchen (with a 'Staff Only' notice on the door) also limit the opportunities for interaction.

Similarly, the physical layout of wards, day rooms, clinics and people's own homes constrains the amount and quality of interaction. It is not surprising to find nurses standing at the foot of the bed to talk to bedridden patients, if all the corridors pass the bed ends. The physical distance that is maintained makes it difficult to have intimate conversations. Day rooms that have the chairs placed round the edges of the room, or facing the television or the window, make it difficult to converse with anyone but an immediate neighbour. This arrangement is typical of many settings for elderly or psychologically disabled people. It is particularly important to understand the limiting effect of the physical layout if part of patient progress is judged by the amount or quality of their interactions (as, for example, in elderly or psychiatric settings). People's own homes can be just as obstructive to good interpersonal relations. Take, for example, the community nurse visiting a middle-aged woman, severely disabled by multiple sclerosis. She is depressed and upset about her own deteriorating physical condition and the effect this is having on her marriage. She does, however, try to keep herself occupied with books and simple handicrafts. As a result, her chair is surrounded by these activities, effectively creating a barrier between herself and anyone else she is talking to. Will it be possible for the nurse to get close enough to her in order to respond warmly or therapeutically? Probably not! Her/his interpersonal skills are curtailed by the physical barrier the patient has constructed around herself. The ways the physical environment can affect the use of interpersonal skills by both nurses and patients are explored in Exercise 9.6.

Exercise 9.6   Environmental constraints on the use of interpersonal skills: physical features

---

Instructions

1. Think of a nursing setting you have worked in recently and draw a map of the setting. Include as many physical features as you can and make some mention of heating, lighting, smells and noise.

Answer sheet

Map of nursing setting: (Type of setting

2. Discuss with a partner how interpersonal skills might be constrained or enhanced in this particular setting, with reference to the discussion issues.

Discussion issues

1. Are demanding patients those that are least accessible?
2. Do nurses try to compensate for the physical setting in terms of their use of interpersonal skills? How?
3. How could you re-design the setting to encourage better use of interpersonal skills by nurses?

Comments

The type of chairs, height of beds and so on may have been noted in Exercise 9.6 as producing certain kinds of interaction. The style and position of furnishings is important too, affecting the feelings of the people using them (and thereby interpersonal skills).

Control over the physical environment

In the course of our everyday lives we have areas of personal and defensible space, space that we can lay claim to, put our personal possessions in and, if we want to, keep other people out of. In hospital there are few ways that people can claim any territory as their own. Furniture can rarely be arranged to create an area of defensible space around a bed; personal effects are few and patients are often discouraged from sticking cards, photos, etc. on their bedsteads. Patients — even long stay patients — rarely have any say over the style of furniture, curtains, etc. It is generally thought that if we are unable to control our physical environment we are liable to experience distress, which in turn will serve to inhibit our usual interpersonal skills. Similarly, if rooms are too hot, too noisy or too smelly and we cannot do anything about this, we may become disgruntled, and in extreme cases experience considerable stress. It is very difficult for nurses (or anyone) to be considerate if they are hot and uncomfortable, have a headache and feel nauseated.

The critical aspect of these environmental constraints is whether or not individual people have any control over them. If for example a particular patient moves the position of her/his bed, so she/he is better able to see out of the window, nurses may well simply move it back again. The patient will learn she/he is not able to determine where her/his bed will go and will feel 'thwarted'. This may end up in a dispute between patient and nurses that would otherwise not have occurred. The nurses, too, by the patient attempting to control his/her environment, may be 'forced' to explain why the bed must stay where it is, what the regulations/rules are, and so on. Thus the content of their interaction with the patient is being determined, indirectly, by the physical environment.

Exercise 9.7 encourages reflection on the physical environment of nursing with a view to identifying those specific features that individual people are unable to control, and that therefore indirectly affect the use of interpersonal skills.

There is another way by which the physical environment affects social behaviour, and that is through what we call the portable environment.

Exercise 9.7 Environmental constraints on the use of the interpersonal skills: thwartings

Instructions

1. Think of a nursing setting you have worked in recently and draw a map of that setting. Include as many features as you can and make some mention of heating, lighting, smells and noise. Use the same map as in Exercise 9.7 if preferred.

Answer sheet

Map of nursing setting: (Type of setting

2. With a partner, identify those features of the environment over which users have no control (decor, temperature, style/position of furniture, clothing, etc.) with reference to the discussion issues.

Discussion issues

1. Might any of these features lead to a feeling of being 'thwarted'? Which?
2. How do feelings of being thwarted affect the interpersonal skills of nurses/patients/relatives? Give examples.
3. Are there any ways these 'thwartings' might be overcome?

Comments

Portable environment

The portable environment refers to those movable features of a setting that tell other people something about the people involved and so go some way to determining how they behave towards these people. Let us take mental health nursing as our example. Clients are often presented to the world in ways that make it difficult for them to be accepted by others as 'ordinary people'. We are all familiar with problems of hospital clothing which frequently seems to carry the message 'this person is a mental patient', perhaps because of half-mast trousers, styles more suited to older or younger people, and so on. Nurses accompanying clients out and about may well act towards them in inappropriate ways, partly as a result of their portable environments. For example the 30-year-old woman with a mental handicap, who is wearing ankle socks and a baggy print dress, may be spoken to as if she were a child. Let us consider too the signs around hospitals (Danger: Patients Walking) or hostels for children with mental handicaps (Slow Children); uncorrected obesity; inappropriate greetings that are encouraged (people with mental handicaps who approach and want to hug complete strangers); phenothiazine gaits, and so on. What does it mean when a local Round Table advertise *'balmy boat race to raise money for handicapped children'*? All these and more conspire to say damaging things about our clients and encourage certain attitudes and prejudices in nurses which constrain their use of interpersonal skill in ways that prohibit their clients from experiencing ordinary relationships.

A good example of how the content of nurse conversation can be affected by the portable environment can be seen in the following (apocryphal) story. Two nurses were taking some clients from a mental handicap hospital on an outing in a minibus. The minibus was a portable environment in so far as it had 'Starlight House: Hospital for the Mentally Handicapped: Donated by Dogooders Business Society' written on the sides. This tells 'outsiders' quite a bit about the occupants both in terms of their disabilities and as objects of charity. One nurse was driving, so *he* could not be a client. The other might have been 'mistaken' for a client, though, so whenever he could, he spoke in such a way as to make it clear that he was *not* mentally handicapped, just in case anyone should be watching/listening to him. The efforts he spent doing this meant that he spent very little time actually talking to the clients. He was acting like this in order to overcome the stigmatizing effects of the portable environment.

These issues do not only relate to the mental health services, they are also relevant to other nursing settings. Health service stickers and community nurses' cars, the wearing of uniforms in the community, bars at the windows of hospitals, etc. are all examples of the portable environment that can affect attitudes and thereby interpersonal skills. Societal attitudes (and nurses are part of society) and values reflect the cultural content of nursing and it is worth stopping for a moment to consider how interpersonal skills are affected by the wider social issues.

9.4 Cultural constraints

At first glance it may seem that the wider social or cultural environment can have little effect on the interpersonal skills of nurses. We will argue, though, that it does, and that the effects are widespread and can be both direct and indirect.

Ideology

We live in a society where the prevailing ideology is one of individual control and responsibility. We are expected (and expect others) to take responsibility for, and to control, all aspects of our lives, including our health. Thus when we find that health is not within our control, the consequences are particularly traumatic and we may find ourselves in a state of 'helplessness' which itself is demoralizing and stressful. It is sometimes argued that physical and psychiatric illness may be a way of coping with other uncontrollable events in our lives. The emphasis on personal responsibility throughout every facet of life puts very real constraints on how nurses relate to other people. Let us take health education for example. Nurses are increasingly expected to fulfil a health educator role (this emphasis is in itself a direct result of policy, stemming from both governmental policies and cultural values). But what kind of health education are they encouraged to promote? It is unlikely that nurses will interpret this role as explaining/informing/teaching members of the public how governmental policies and environmental issues can have direct consequences on everybody's health. It is, instead, more likely that they will interpret it as explaining/informing/teaching people how they can eat, exercise, drink, look after themselves (such as the Health Education Council's propaganda scheme called 'Look After Yourself'), etc. so that their chances of enjoying good health are increased. Given this orientation, nurses will use particular interpersonal skills in pursuit of particular goals. Thus, ideology both directly affects nurses' use of interpersonal skills and indirectly affects them via governmental and professional policies.

It is worth considering what happens to the nurse when she/he meets someone who flatly refuses to follow the advice/recommendations. The nurse may experience conflict because another ideological force operating is that of the importance of choice and the exercise of free will. We like to think we do have choice over different aspects of our lives, but in reality we may find we do not. Nurses may experience problems in relating to people who *do* exercise free choice in ways that go directly against the nurse's personal stance. As nurses are both suppliers and (potential) consumers of health care, it may be useful to ask at such times 'What would *I* do, or how would *I* feel in such circumstances?'

The 'freedom of choice' issue leads into the ethical and moral contexts of nursing. Nurses who try to exercise their free choice over ethical/moral issues may find themselves in direct conflict with colleagues or indeed their professional bodies. A recent example of this is the nurse who refuses to participate in giving electro-convulsive shock treatment because she/he believes it is morally wrong, and at the same time believes that she/he is entitled to work within her/his moral framework. The interpersonal skills she/he will have to use with colleagues and/or management will be those of assertion, negotiation, and possibly confrontation. If it were not for the conflicting pressures, these particular interpersonal events might not take place. It may be useful, here, to look again at Exercise 2.4 which explored different kinds of beliefs about nursing. Which of these beliefs may lead to the type of conflict described above, and possibly, in turn, to *interpersonal* conflict?

We have seen, then, that ideology can directly curtail the interpersonal skills of nurses. It can also have indirect effects in so far as it helps determine (and is determined by) government policies and attitudes towards health care, and these in turn affect nurses' interpersonal relationships.

Government policies

The policies of different governments towards health care, and in particular the role that the National Health Service (NHS) is to play in the delivery of that care, can affect nurses in several ways, with implications for their use of interpersonal skills. The funding of the NHS has consequences for staffing levels and hence the opportunities to talk with patients as well as for nurses' morale. Cuts in specific health services might make it very difficult for a nurse to reply honestly to a patient's plea, 'Can nothing be done?' This is especially so when she/he believes that there may have been some hope, if the specialist service had not been cut. These types of effects are different for different care groups, as priority areas are identified. Current policies supporting 'care in the community' systems will affect both the status of the health services (as opposed to social services) and require that more nurses employ their interpersonal skills in community settings. Restructuring the NHS has effects on nurses' morale every time it occurs, as they are repeatedly asked to work in the context of considerable personal insecurity.

The growth of privatization of health care, and the support given to the pharmaceutical industry both help to create a tension in the need to make profits out of health care. Nurses may find themselves compromised in various ways or subject to massive advertising and propaganda campaigns which restrict their decision-making processes, and may well then influence what advice they give patients (although of course, we all like to believe that we are not open to such influences!).

There are many other ways that government policies can have an effect on the interpersonal skills of nurses, but these examples should serve to illustrate the point. Both government and prevailing ideologies influence the professional bodies concerned with nursing.

Professional nursing bodies

It is the professional nursing bodies that prescribe the role of the nurse in the general and specific training syllabi for the various specialisms. Thus they determine the professional attitude towards the importance of interpersonal skills, and hence the amount of time spent in training and serious consideration that should be paid to these aspects of nursing. Currently, the English National Board and the United Kingdom Central Council for Nursing and Midwifery and Health Visiting all concede the importance of interpersonal skill as a vital nursing skill. Nevertheless, the relative importance varies with the type of nursing. A glance at the different syllabi will reveal the relative importance given to interpersonal issues. A look too at examination papers over the years will reveal a changing emphasis with regard to interpersonal skills, but it is still interesting to see the amount of emphasis given to interpersonal issues in comparison with other nursing skills, and the degree to which different courses outline the *specific*

Exercise 9.8   Cultural constraints on the use of interpersonal skills

---

Instructions

Please choose one of the mass media (television, radio, newspapers, women's magazines, films, etc.) and examine it for references to health, illness and nursing. What does this tell you about the cultural context in which nursing takes place? Ask the following questions:

Answer sheet

1. *How are nurses represented?* (As policy-makers/doctors' assistants/not at all in their own right, etc.)

2. *What attitude towards health/illness is presented?* (Individual/societal responsibility; controllable/not, etc.)

3. *What role of government is stated or implied?*

4. *What topics of illness are mentioned, and with what frequency?* (Frequently/occasionally/never)

5. *What comparisons are made with other health care systems?* (In other countries/at other times etc.)

6. *Who will be seeing/reading/listening to this source of information?*

7. *Are different 'messages' presented for different audiences/readers? (How?)*

8. *Are references to women, men, children, people from different age/cultural groups different? (In what ways?)*

9. *How much of the total space/time is devoted to these issues?*

Describe the expectations and pressures that surround nursing, based on what you have seen, heard or read.

Consider the implications of this analysis with reference to the discussion issues.

Discussion issues

1. How do government policies influence practical nursing directly/indirectly?
2. Are there any taboo topics in this society to do with health/illness? What are they and how have they come about?

3. What happens if nurses blur the distinction between private and professional roles? Is this used by the media?
4. What role do nurses have in bringing about political/social change?

Variations: Examine your media source over time: look at the popular nursing press at 5-year intervals for changes in the view of nurses/nursing. Examine the same materials as a partner and compare notes.

Comments

---

interpersonal skills to be acquired. If the training bodies do not place interpersonal skills high on their list of priorities, why should other practising nurses or nurses in training?.

In this section, we have discussed some of the features of the social or cultural context of nursing which can impose direct or indirect constraints on nurses' use of interpersonal skills. Some ideas for developing further awareness of these issues are given in Exercise 9.8.

It is only with such awareness that nurses can realistically understand and appraise their own interpersonal skills, a notion that further supports the need for all nurses to work towards increasing their own self-awareness as we have argued in Chapter 2.

9.5 Summary

This chapter has focused on the context of interpersonal skills used by nurses. Specifically, the following points were raised:

The effective use of interpersonal skill depends on the personal, social, environmental and cultural contexts in which they are deployed.

In order to overcome the constraints imposed by the context of nursing, nurses must learn to recognize them.

Nurses are increasingly expected to contact patients at an emotional level which inevitably arouses their own emotions.

Stress and low morale may result from increased emotional involvement with patients.

Emotion, stress and low morale may all distort the use of interpersonal skills.

Intimate relationships between nurses and patients develop in particular ways that differ from the development of other relationships.

Personal support systems should help alleviate the levels of stress experienced by nurses.

The interaction context in part determines the scope of interpersonal skills.

Patients (playing sick roles) put demands on nurses' interpersonal skills.

Regulations prescribe implicitly and/or explicitly a range of interpersonal skills.

Organizational factors constrain both the opportunities for and channels of effective interpersonal relations.

Bureaucratic tasks reduce the time available to talk with patients.

Organizational climate contributes to the level of morale experienced by nurses and indirectly their use of interpersonal skill.

Organizational climate is perceived differently by people at different stages of their careers.

Physical environments can directly inhibit the use of particular interpersonal skills.

Physical factors can limit the opportunities for interaction.

Lack of control over physical features of the environment can lead to stress.

Portable environments help determine and maintain attitudes and prejudices and indirectly affect the nature and use of interpersonal skills.

Cultural ideology constrains nurses' use of interpersonal skills, both directly and indirectly, via government policies.

Ideology surrounds the ethical and moral dilemmas faced by nurses and these can have indirect consequences for their use of interpersonal skills.

Governmental policies and attitudes towards health care influence nurses' morale and thereby their effective use of interpersonal skills.

Government and prevailing ideology influence professional nursing bodies which in turn prescribe the status given to interpersonal skills in nursing.

Further reading

Beardshaw, V. (1981) *Conscientious Objectors at Work: Mental Hospital Nurses — A Case Study*, Social Audit, London

Doyle, L. (1979) *The Politics of Health*, Pluto Press, London

Gow, K.M. (1982) *How Nurses' Emotions Affect Patient Care*, Springer, New York

Jacobson, S.F. (1983) The contexts of nurses' stress. In S.F. Jacobson and H.M. McGrath (Eds.) *Nurses Under Stress*, Wiley, New York

Kagan, C. (Ed.) (1985) The context of interpersonal skills, *Interpersonal Skills in Nursing: Research and Applications*, Croom Helm, London, Section III

Kalisch, P.A., Kalisch, B.J. and Scobey, M. (1983) *Images of Nurses in Television*, Springer, New York

Salvage, J. (1985) *The Politics of Nursing*, Heinemann, London

Smith, V.M. and Bass, T.A. (1982) You and the organization, *Communication for the Health Care Team*, Harper and Row, London, Ch. 10

CHAPTER 10

COMPLEX SOCIAL ROUTINES

In previous sections we have introduced the idea that many social situations have rituals associated with them. Rituals are taken to be recurring patterns of behaviour linked to the roles that people occupy and the social rules they follow. In Chapter 4 we explored two fundamental social rituals, namely those of interaction openings and closures. Complex interactions too have ritualistic aspects, as we have seen throughout this book. It is useful to explore some complex nursing interactions, both to practise the skills introduced in previous sections and to gain insight into the thoughts, feelings and actions of other people involved, whether they be patients, relatives, colleagues or other professionals. Role play and simulation games offer valuable opportunities to experience complex social situations out of context in what would, hopefully, be a safe and non-threatening environment.

10.1 Role play and simulation games

Role play and simulation games require examination of the ritualistic aspects of interaction. Both allow for the manipulation of the roles and rules associated with particular situations. Many of the exercises included in this book have used basic role play techniques. Some have required students to engage in *passive* role play (for example, Exercises 4.3 and 4.4 that ask students to *imagine* what they might say if they were nurses in various situations), and some in *active* role play (for example, Exercises 8.4 and 8.5 that ask students to adopt roles of 'clients' and 'counsellor'). Passive role play then requires students to think and relate how they might act in a particular role in a particular situation. Active role play is the stronger form and enables students to have some direct experience of the forces surrounding specific roles in specific situations.

Simulations and games are often extended and complex role plays. They are structured to include background information about resources, constraints, goals and rules as well as about activities of the 'players'. They are frequently used to develop problem solving skills and as a means of demonstrating the effects of positive and negative attitudes.

Advantages of using role play or simulation techniques

Whilst both role play and simulation techniques can be valuable, we do have some reservations in their use: thus advantages should be seen in the light of the disadvantages.

Both active role play and simulation allow students to experiment with new behaviour in a non-threatening environment: they can practise and change behaviour without having to worry about 'getting it wrong'. If some of the roles that are used are familiar ones, students may be able to identify their personal behaviour patterns. This can be surprising (sometimes shocking!) and may lead participants to work towards changing some aspects of their behaviour. Change may also result from the increased awareness and sensitivity that is gained if opportunity for constructive and realistic feedback is offered (see next section). It is often argued that such increased awareness is the major advantage of role play and simulation. The awareness need not be limited to self-awareness. Through experience, participants will also become aware of pressures that exist in the creation of roles, whether they be roles that are adopted by individuals themselves or imposed by others. It can be quite illuminating to discover the demands and expectations impinging upon us in our different roles and perhaps most importantly, how other people (involved in the role play) interpret these pressures.

Awareness of the rules that underlie and constraints that operate to limit particular roles may also follow from involvement in role play or simulation. Whenever students are asked to act out roles they are unfamiliar with, they acquire some direct experience of what it is like to be in this new role. Whilst people differ with regard to the ease with which they can 'take the role of the other', techniques of role reversal (whereby participants exchange roles and repeat an exercise) do encourage the growth of empathy. The ways in which participants' role partners interpret and act their own roles, will lead them to question their own interpretations and to develop a wider range of problem solving skills. This is one of the reasons why role play and simulation are often used to enhance problem solving skills.

In addition to providing opportunities for direct experience, role play and simulation provide facilities for participants to receive feedback about their interpretations and performances. This feedback is critical in deriving maximum learning benefit from role play experiences. Figure 10.1 summarizes the active role playing process.

Feedback

The feedback participants get from role play and simulations can vary in terms of its subjectivity and objectivity. On one level, all participants get some feedback from their role partners in the course of the role play. They can assess their own performances in the light of how others are performing. When the role play is completed, discussion between all those involved substantiates this feedback. Such discussions are an integral part of any role play and should never be excluded: it is quite dissatisfying for those involved to miss the chance to share their feelings and understanding of what was going on during the role play.

A less subjective form of feedback can be given by other people who have watched the role play. They may have watched it directly, either in the same room or through a one-way mirror. They may also have watched a film or heard a recording of the role play, in other words have observed indirectly. Whichever way, observers' perceptions and interpretations of the performance will probably offer new insights to the participants. Observing and exploring other people's role plays can be a valuable experience in its own right and observers can develop awareness and sensitivity without the direct experiences.

The least subjective form of feedback is gained from watching/hearing video/audio tapes of the performance. The advantage of (particularly) video tape is that viewers can see what really happened: that is, what participants really did and said. Video tape cannot, however, reveal the social effects of what was done/said. In other words, it cannot give any information of how interaction partners felt or thought about a particular player's performance.

Figure 10.1 Active role play

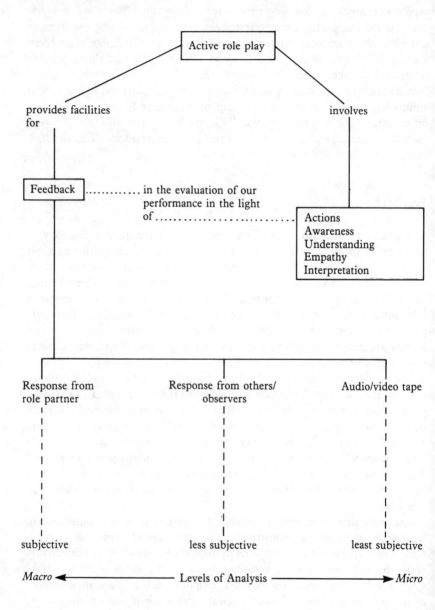

This is an important point to bear in mind as a video tape can distort social reality. The importance of different facets of behaviour can be over-emphasized on film so that actions seem to be wanting on film are quite acceptable in reality. This means that discussion of the films by all those participating (and perhaps others as well) are essential if the performances are to be put in some realistic context.

Having said this, though, there is no doubt that video-taped feedback is invaluable for the examination of the minutiae of social performance (non-verbal and verbal components) and in confronting participants with images of themselves. It is sometimes argued that such micro-analysis derived from video-taped confrontation is the most efficient way of precipitating both behaviour change and self-awareness.

We cannot stress too strongly the importance of constructive monitoring and processing of all forms of feedback is, particularly video-taped feedback. Some people 'seeing themselves as others see them' for the first time are shocked at their appearance and how they sound, and, seemingly, at the gross inadequacies of their interaction skills. They become so preoccupied with self-criticism that it is difficult for them to extract anything positive from the experience. These people are likely to become distressed at their performance, a reaction that can lead to lack of confidence, embarrassment and anxiety with concomitant consequences for their effective use of interpersonal skill. Such reactions can be minimized by careful, sensitive processing of the video tapes by all concerned. If this is done, video-taped feedback can certainly lead to personal growth and behaviour change.

Disadvantages of using role play and simulation techniques

We mentioned above that some students react adversely to video-taped feedback. Similarly, some students find the whole role play/simulation acitivity extremely anxiety provoking. This anxiety can be ameliorated to a certain extent by careful preparation and introduction by tutors. As with all experiential methods, no students should be asked to do anything they do not want to do. However, if some students persistently refuse to become involved in role plays they will not only be missing valuable learning opportunities but will also be exploiting the willingness of more confident colleagues. Contracting (see Chapter 1) and discussion with individual students may help overcome their worries. Nevertheless, the onus for constructive processing of all role play performances will usually lie with tutors and they should be confident that they are able to do this before engaging in role play.

Tutors should also be confident that they can handle distress in the classroom if they are using role plays that are likely to elicit strong reactions from the actors (and this is not always easy to anticipate). Students can become engrossed in their role, and may be surprised at the strengths of their own reactions to what is, after all, 'only a game'. It can be seen, then, that role play, perhaps more than other experiential methods included in this book, requires a breakdown of formal tutor–student relationships. Tutors are not in the position of judging performances in role plays, but rather of facilitating insights through guiding, interpreting, inspiring and stimulating students.

We mentioned, above that video-taped feedback can be distorting. So, too can the entire role play experience. This is due to the role plays frequently compressing time and thereby distorting experiences. Again, though, careful processing can alleviate the effects of this.

Role plays may seem to be divorced from reality. Whilst they offer the opportunity to sample the real world in a risk-free environment, this chance is missed if the links between the role play and reality are poorly drawn. Students may think that the exercise was stupid and have difficulty generalizing their experiences to real life situations. Once again it is the level of tutor's skills that will determine the value of the learning experience for students.

Even though most role plays can be made simple, they are very demanding on time. If they are to run smoothly, quite considerable preparation must be done and clear instruction given to participants so that they treat the sessions seriously (see Section 10.2). Table 10.1 summarizes the advantages and disadvantages of role play and simulation techniques.

Despite the disadvantages of using role play and simulation techniques, if properly organized, we believe they do increase student motivation and heighten interest and excitement in learning for most people. There are, however, some considerations to be made when planning and implementing role play and simulation sessions.

Table 10.1   Role play and simulation techniques: advantages and disadvantages

---

Advantages
Heighten interest and excitement in learning
Encourage identification of personal behaviour patterns, possibly leading to change
Allow participants to experiment with new behaviours in a risk free environment
Increase awareness and sensitivity, possibly leading to change
Provide insights into attitudes and values
Facilitate the development of empathy by providing opportunities to 'take the role of the other'
Offer the chance to experience the pressures of creating roles (i.e. demands and expectations)
Give insights into the rules of adopting particular roles and of the constraints that limit their expression.
Encourage the development of problem-solving skills
Provide opportunities for receiving feedback at a variety of levels
Challenge traditional tutor-student relationships

Disadvantages
Unfamiliar to students and teachers, possibly leading to anxiety and distrust
Full involvement in a role may lead to student distress
Some students may refuse to participate
Some students may not take the activities seriously
Tutors need skills to facilitate the development of insight
Feedback can be traumatic and must be handled with sensitivity
It may be difficult to ensure that the links with real life situations are clear and meaningful
Time consuming and often misunderstood by colleagues

10.2 Implementation of role play and simulation techniques

Student anxieties

If role plays are to be taken seriously, students should not be coerced into taking part. Reluctant participants will perform unenthusiastically and limit the learning opportunities for others. It is usually essential to give some clarification concerning the role plays to students. Student anxiety may be somewhat reduced if they are told:

(a) The purpose of role play is to provide participants with insights and opportunities to practise (possibly) new behaviours in situations they may not have met before. The idea is to practise the behaviours in a risk-free environment before trying them out in the real situation.

(b) Role-played behaviours will not be judged. Instead they will be discussed constructively.

(c) There are no right and wrong ways to interpret and perform different roles. However, the discussions may well consider alternative ways they could have been enacted.

It is not assumed that people act in role plays as they do in real life situations. Whilst every attempt is made to ensure that role plays resemble reality, only the participants themselves will know how closely their own performance resembled their real life behaviour.

Above all else, the purpose of a particular role play should be disclosed, at the start if possible, or else during the processing of the session. Discussion should consider how well the role play met its objectives and tutors should be open to constructive criticism. In this way, tutors will be setting an example of open tutor-student relationships.

Students may also have anxieties *after* doing their role plays. Tutors must be able to pick these up and ensure that adequate time is left to discuss the concerns in class, or individually as appropriate. If necessary participants should be de-roled. (see Practical Issues section below.)

Preparation

Role plays and simulations are analogous to theatrical performances. Their preparation, therefore, require scenes to be set, characters to be drawn and scripts to be written. The amount of detail given to the actors will depend on their previous experiences and familiarity with the parts they are to play. Thus it may be sufficient to say to some students that 'the encounter takes place in a cubicle off Nightingale ward between a patient who is having an ECG and a qualified nurse'. Other students may need a full description of the ward, the electrocardiogram procedure and extent of patient immobility, as well as likely biographical information about the patient and the nurse, depending on how much knowledge of such situations can be assumed. Even with limited experience, though, role playing in the light of little information can reveal actors' stereotypes of the parts they are playing and can, therefore, be useful. The amount of information that is given will depend, too, on the extent to which participants are to interpret the role and the situation for themselves. If extensive interpretation is wanted, relatively little information should be given. In these cases, students often ask for more detail and should be told to interpret as best they can on the basis of the information they have been given.

Role plays can also vary according to the features typifying a role analysis of social behaviour (see Chapter 4). Thus role strain may be introduced to a particular role or conflict between roles aroused. The demands made on a particular role may be clearly outlined or left ambiguous. Similarly, each actor may be told of other's expectations of her/him or they may have to assume these. Lastly, the rules associated with the scene and/or the role(s) may be made explicit, or they too may be left to be assumed.

Generally, simulations are more tightly scripted, with background information about the situation and the characters, resources, goals, constraints and activities all being included. They are frequently used for management training, but there is no reason why they should not be used at all levels of interpersonal skills training. They are, however, time consuming, and great care must be taken to ensure that their relevance to real life is made quite clear.

Practical issues

The part of the audience should be defined, and at the very least the following questions should be considered: Will observers watch the role play from the same room or through a one-way screen? If the role play is to be video taped, will everyone watch it with or without the actors being present? What guidelines relating to constructive discussion of the scenarios, and of ensuring confidentiality of the proceedings will be issued? How can observers be encouraged to be as unobtrusive as possible, so as not to interrupt the performance? It is as important for observers to treat the exercise seriously as it is for actors to.

As with all interpersonal skills work, role plays require careful thought about the suitability of the settings in which they take place. Some of the most important questions to ask are: Is the room big enough? Are any props (such as beds for 'patients') needed and available? If the role plays are to be video taped can this be done unobtrusively?

Some students get very involved with their role(s) and may find it difficult to step out of them at the end of the session. This is particularly likely if the role(s) contain emotional elements or if the progress of the role play leads to emotional encounters. Sometimes role enactment can trigger previous emotional experiences for some students. Tutors may, at times, have to call a premature halt to a role play if the extent of emotionality is likely to be destructive. When intense role enactment has occurred, tutors should ensure that participants are de-roled. Discussion of experiences helps to do this, but it can sometimes be necessary to ask students to state who and where they are. If all participants do this, no one person will feel stupid or embarrassed. Tutors should be alert to the possiblity that individual students may need further time to de-role after the session.

10.3 Sample role plays

In this section we will give some examples of role plays that vary in terms of their objectives, intensity, detail, and manipulation of features of a role analysis of social behaviour. Variations of Exercises 10.1–10.4 can be devised to meet particular individual and class needs.

Exercise 10.1 The experience of dependency

Objective

To gain insight into the experience of being dependent on another person.

Instructions

Choose any state of dependency. With a partner, act out the roles of *'helper'* and *'dependant'*. Follow the guidelines.

Guidelines

Before beginning your role play, establish the following:

1. How long will the role play last? (Stick to the agreed time.)
2. What will you do if one of the roles 'breaks down'? (Terminate role play/carry on etc.?)
3. How much time will be available for discussion at the end?
4. Will you discuss your roles before starting, or allow them to develop spontaneously?

If you need to add to your role script, draw on your personal experience to do so. At the end of the role play, share your experiences in the light of the discussion issues. Examples of low and high dependency role plays are given below.

Low Dependency

Blindness

With a partner, allocate roles A — blind person and B — sighted person.
Activity: Blindfold A. For 1 hour, continue with everyday activities together — shopping, eating in canteen, walking around the buildings, etc. Establish some guidelines (for example, can the blind person speak/hear? Do you know each other well? etc.) Try not to discuss the experience until the alloted time is up. At the end of the role play, share your experiences in the light of the discussion issues.

Discussion issues

1. What struck you most about the role you played?
2. Would you have behaved differently if your partner had been a stranger? How/why?
3. Can you imagine what it would have been like if you had to play these roles for a full week?

High dependency

Stroke/mental handicap

With a partner, allocate roles A — person with stroke or a mental handicap, and B — nurse.

Activity: Go to a canteen or a cafe for a meal. If you can, choose a venue where there will be other people that you know. A — sit at the table. You cannot speak nor move your arms or head. B — you have the responsibility for seeing that the meal goes smoothly. A will need feeding. At the end of the meal, share your experiences in the light of the discussion issues.

Discussion issues

1. Did B try to ascertain A's preferences? If so, what problems arose? If not, why not?
2. Would A have preferred B to act differently? How?
3. How did you feel doing this activity with other people around that you knew?
4. Would you have felt differently if your partner had been a stranger/10 years older/from a different cultural background? Why?
5. What must it be like to be permanently in a state of high dependence?

Comments

Exercise 10.2   Simple role enactment and role reversal

Objectives

To practise some likely aspects of the nursing role and gain insight into the role of patient/relative through role reversal.

Instructions

With a partner, act out the following roles. Spend ten minutes on each scenario. Do not discuss your roles before doing the role play. Draw on your personal experience to 'add' to the role scripts. After each role play discuss the discussion issues.

Reassuring anxious relative

Situation

Coronary care unit (CCU) of large district general hospital. Victor Jones was admitted to the CCU three days ago, and was making satisfactory progress. Just before being moved to the medical ward he has a cardiac arrest and is successfully resuscitated, although he is still ill. His wife was telephoned when he was taken ill and has arrived at the unit door. Staff nurse tells the third-year student nurse to take Mrs Jones to a side ward for a cup of tea while she waits for the doctor.

Roles

Third-year student nurse explaining what has happened.
Mrs Jones, a 52-year-old woman, married for 34 years.

Talking with a distressed patient

Situation

Mrs Dawn Cartwright is aged 35 years and works as a fashion model for a mail-order catalogue. One week ago she found a lump in her left breast. She has now been admitted for surgery and there is a possibility of a left simple mastectomy.

Roles

Mrs Cartwright.
Second-year student nurse talking to her about the forthcoming surgery.

Talking with a belligerent, recently bereaved relative

Situation

Mr Albert Hughes, 38 years, was admitted to the medical unit at 7 p.m. in an extremely ill state, in severe left ventricular failure. He was accompanied by his wife who left after visiting time. Mr Hughes died during the night. His wife was telephoned but did not wish to come to the hospital at that time. She now arrives at the ward at about 10 a.m. and demands to know the whereabouts of an expensive electric razor which she says her husband brought in with him.

Roles

Staff nurse dealing with this siuation.

Mrs Hughes, aged 37 years, two children ages 8, 10, previously worked as a clerical assistant in an insurance office. There is money still owing on the mortgage and Mr Hughes has cashed his life insurance policy on being made redundant eighteen months ago.

Talking with an emotional patient on discharge

Situation

Mrs Barker, aged 42 years, personal secretary to bank manager, is being discharged from hospital following a hysterectomy for fibroids (her ovaries have been conserved). While awaiting her husband, she becomes tearful, claiming that she will not be able to cope at home with either her domestic, work or private life. Whilst in hospital, she annoyed other patients by telling them how they should rearrange their lives in order to avoid 'cracking up'. The staff nurse is talking to her.

Roles

Staff Nurse. You are the only trained nurse on duty — the E.N. (G.) is off sick and your colleague has been transferred to another ward that is even more short-staffed for the day. You did not enjoy nursing Mrs Barker.

Mrs Barker

Discussion issues

1. How easy was it to play the role of (a) nurse, (b) patient/relative?
2. What insights did you gain through role reversal? What did it feel like to play the patient/relative?
3. Have you ever found yourself in a similar situation? If so, please describe what happened? Did you deal with the 'real' situation differently from the role-played situation? In what ways?
4. How would the role play have differed if your role was of the opposite sex? Why is it difficult to role play the opposite sex?
5. Did this role play fulfil the objectives of the exercises? Can you think of any ways those objectives might be better met?

Comments

Exercise 10.3 Role conflict through differing expectations and excessive demands

-----

Objectives

1. To experience role conflict that arises through differing expectations.
2. To devise some strategies for handling role conflict due to differing expectations.
3. To gain insight into some of the stresses caused by unreasonable demands.

Instructions

With a partner, act out the following roles. Spend 10 minutes on each scenario. Do not discuss your roles before doing the role play. After each role play consider the discussion issues. As the role plays rely on each person not knowing the expectations brought by her/his partner, the role scripts for person A are given below. Person B will find her/his role scripts on pp. 334–37. Draw on your personal experience to 'add' to the role scripts.

The 'rights' of elderly people (1)

Person A — Elderly patient

A — you are Mrs Gertrude Campbell, aged 76. You live alone in a neat one-bedroomed flat, and are quite happy. Your daughter and her family visit regularly. You are having increasing difficutly with your vision, which you put down to growing old. Reluctantly you have seen the doctor who tells you she wants to operate. You do not want surgery as you believe this entails 'having your eye taken out'. You are terrified of hospitals and want to be left in peace. Your daughter thinks you are entitled to your own views. She has told you that the community nurse will be able to support you in your arguments with the doctor.

Task

You aim to convince the nurse you do not want surgery.

The 'rights' of elderly people (2)

Person A — Staff nurse

A — you are about to discharge Mr Green, age 67, following a hip replacement. He has been difficult and unpleasant to nurse. He is surly, disparaging and bad tempered. At the same time, he tries to do little for himself, being quite content to be 'waited on' in hospital. Before the ambulance arrives, you are just clarifying with him the arrangements with the district nursing service so that some continuity of care is maintained when he goes home. You know from his records that his home is messy and that it smells. He has three cats that are not well tended.

Task

You aim to clarify the arrangement for home nursing.

Conflicting concerns

Person A — Patient

A — you are a 42-year-old woman who has been admitted to hospital for 'investigations' concerning a recurrent stomach problem. You have had a good deal of discomfort for several years now and the GP has not been able to treat you successfully. You have been assured that the investigations are routine and will not entail anything unpleasant. You are a little apprehensive as you have not been in hospital before, but your main concern is how your two teenage children will manage at home by themselves whilst you are in hospital.

Task

You want to check the details for your stay so you can reassure yourself that your arrangements have been satisfactory

Professional rivalry

Person A — Staff nurse

A — you are a new (male) staff nurse appointed to work on an understaffed children's ward. One of the regular staff is a S.E.N. who has been working on this ward for 14 years. She is a good bit older and more experienced than you. However much you wish to be pleasant to her and to learn from her, you find her constant belligerent 'holier than thou' attitude difficult to combat. Recently the nursing management has been keen to emphasize the policy of two trained staff to administer drugs. This does not include S.E.N.s. In the absence of the ward sister one afternoon, you have to insist that the S.E.N. does not take part in the drug round.

Task

You try to make her see that she cannot take part in the drug round.

Professional boundaries

Person A — Student nurse

A — you are a second-year student nurse on a general medical ward (male). One of the patients, Mr Foster, has formed quite an attachment to you. You enjoy nursing him, as he is always in good spirits and has a good supply of jokes. He has had no visitors during the three weeks he has been in, although his records show that he has some close family living nearby. You have often told him, jokingly, that you would do anything for him — he has only to ask. Today he has asked you to call on his daughter and ask her to come and see him in hospital. You are sure that this would be going beyond the bounds of your professional relationship.

Task

To refuse his request.

Competing roles

Person A — Patient on psychiatric admission ward

A — you are a young woman (20 years old) who has been admitted to a psychiatric ward for the fifth time in three years. You are in a confused state and have recently had some psychotic incidents. At the moment you believe you are taking part in a television show — one of those that play tricks on people to see how well they can 'take a joke'. The nurse that comes to talk to you is one of a close circle of friends, none of whom know you have been in hospital before. You think this is very funny and quite clever of the television company. At the same time you are relieved that one of your friends has 'found out' that you are involved with the hospital.

Task

You feel the need to reassure your friend that you do not mind being involved in the 'joke' nor that your secret has been uncovered.

Personal limitations

Person A — Student nurse

A — you are a student nurse on your first general medical block. You have come on duty on a Saturday morning to find that the ward is short staffed. The only empty bed on the ward was filled last night by a young mother of three who had taken an overdose. The sister says that she would not normally ask such an inexperienced nurse to be responsible for 'such patients', but will have to ask you today, because of the staffing levels. She therefore asks that you pay particular attention to this patient (the ward tries to implement the nursing process and provide individualized patient care). You are apprehensive as you firmly believe in the sanctity of life (you would not be a nurse if you did not), and are a little afraid of 'such patients'.

Task

You take the patient her wash bowl, and try to find out if she needs to go to the toilet.

Resource limitations

Person A — Mrs Barnett

A — you are a 48-year-old woman, severely disabled with multiple sclerosis and confined to a wheelchair. You live in a specially converted flat. It is midsummer and very hot: the flat has inadequate ventilation. The district nurse, who has been coming to visit you for some time, and with whom you have a good relationship, has come to give you your weekly bath. You feel you need daily baths in hot weather and are sure that the nurse will agree to this.

Task

Negotiate over the bath issue.

Discussion issues

1. What were A and B trying to achieve?
2. What strategies did both A and B use? Were they successful strategies? Why/why not?
3. What conflict did each person feel, and how did these affect the way she/he handled the situation?
4. Have you ever met any similar situations at work? If so, what happened?
5. Can you suggest any other ways either A or B might have handled the situation?
6. What was it like playing this role? What insights did the role play produce?

Comments

Exercise 10.4 Ethical dilemmas

Objective

To examine the decision-making process when ethical and moral conflicts arise.

Instructions

With a partner, act out the following roles. Do not put a time limit on each scenario — take as long as you need in order to reach an acceptable conclusion. You may look at each other's role script before beginning, but do not discuss how you will play the role. After each role play, consider the discussion issues. Draw on your personal experience to 'add' to the role scripts.

Issues surrounding the cessation of treatment

Person A — Elderly patient

A — you are Mrs Emma Crawford, age 80 years. You have been ill for two years with what you know is chronic leukaemia. You have undergone cytotoxic therapy which you found distressing although you appreciate that it has prolonged your life. You have just been re-admitted for further blood tests and the physician wishes to start you again on chemotherapy. You are tired and feel enough is enough. You do not wish to see your family suffer any more. Staff Nurse Knight, who you like and trust, enters your side ward. You ask her advice.

Person B — Staff nurse

B — you are Staff Nurse Knight. You have looked after Mrs Crawford for two years, intermittently. You like her and admire her courage. However, when you enter her room, Mrs Crawford appears extremely upset and asks your advice about whether she should continue with the treatment which you feel will only give her a few more weeks at the most.

Issues surrounding the possibility of having a handicapped child

Person A — Pregnant woman

A — you are a woman of 38 years who is 16 weeks pregnant with your second child. You have been trying to conceive for four years and you and your husband were pleased that you had succeeded. You had agreed, reluctantly, to an amniocentesis as your age made the possibility of an abnormality in the development of the fetus quite high (certainly within the health authority's 'risk' category). The amniocentesis indicated fetal abnormality, and the antenatal staff have offered you an abortion. Your husband has said that the decision must be yours, although he has been supportive and has talked through the issues with you. You are still undecided, and would like to talk to the sister in the antenatal clinic, as you have confidence in her experience of such matters.

Person B — Sister in antenatal clinic

B — you are sister in charge of a busy inner city antenatal clinic. You have known Mrs Watts since her first pregnancy six years ago. You know she has been trying for a second baby for some time and that she was pleased to be pregnant. Mrs Watts reluctantly had an amniocentesis, which was positive, and she has been offered an abortion. You believe strongly that a woman's life should come before a (unborn) child's. Even though you know of some families who have gained a great deal from the birth of a mentally handicapped child, you are also aware of the enormous pressure they place on the parents, particularly the mothers. Mrs Watts has asked to see you in order to help her arrive at a decision.

Discussion Issues

1. What were A and B trying to achieve, and why?
2. What strategies did both A and B use? Were they successful strategies? Why/why not?
3. What conflicts did A and B feel and how did this affect the way she/he handled the situation?
4. Have you ever met any similar situations at work? If so, what happened?
5. Can you suggest any other ways either A or B might have handled the situation?
6. What was it like playing this role? What insights did the role play produce?

Comments

10.4 Summary

In this chapter we have discussed the use and implementation of role play and simulation techniques to explore complex social routines of nurses. Specifically the following issues were raised:

Complex interactions may have ritualistic aspects, that is recurring patterns of behaviour linked to the roles that people occupy and the rules they follow.

Role play and simulation techniques provide opportunities to experience complex social situations in a safe, non-threatening environment.

Role play and simulation techniques allow for the manipulation of the roles and rules associated with particular situations.

Active role play requires students to express a role and is a stronger learning experience than passive role play.

Simulations are more highly structured than role plays although they generally include role-played activity.

Role play and simulation have advantages and disadvantages.

Role play may lead to attitude and/or behaviour change.

Role play can lead to increased awareness into the creation and maintenance of roles and the expectations and demands that are brought to bear on them.

Awareness of the rules underlying roles and the constraints that limit their expression may follow role-played experiences.

Role plays offer opportunities to 'take the role of the other' and to develop empathy.

Feedback is an essential component of role play techniques and varies in degree of subjectivity.

Observers of role plays may also gain enhanced awareness and sensitivity.

Video-taped feedback can be traumatic and should be processed with care.

Tutors and students all have a responsibility to ensure that feedback is handled constructively.

Students may be reluctant to participate in role-played sessions and tutors should try to ameliorate their anxieties.

Role play can lead to intense involvement in the role, which can result in the arousal of emotions.

Tutors should be confident in their ability to defuse emotionally charged role plays.

Role plays can distort reality and care must be taken to ensure that relevant links with real life situations are established.

Role plays and simulations are demanding on time and resources.

Role play and simulations increase student motivation by heightening interest and excitement in learning.

Practical considerations relating to student anxieties, necessary preparation and conducting the role plays should be considered.

Role plays can vary in several ways, and the learning objectives should be made clear at the start and finish of each session.

Tutors must be prepared to be open and receive constructive criticism about the role plays from the participants.

Further reading

Brandes, D. and Phillips, H (1977) *Gamesters' Handbook,* Hutchinson, London

Clark, C.C. (1978) *Classroom Skills for Nurse Educators,* Springer, New York

French, H.P. (1980) A place for simulation in nurse education, *Nursing Focus,* July, pp 445–46

Satow, A. and Evans, M. (1983) *Working with Groups,* TACADE, Manchester

van Ments, M. (1983) *The Effective Use of Role Play: A Handbook for Teachers and Trainers,* Kogan Page, London

Williams, L.V. (1978) Patient role play by learners, *Nursing Times,* vol. 4, pp 1402–6

CONCLUSION

Reflections on material that is included

This postscript gives us the opportunity to reflect on the material we have covered, and to consider that which we have not. It also enables us to point to some of the directions we think interpersonal skills for nurses will take in the near future.

At the beginning of the book, we hoped to be able to excite you, the reader and, hopefully, the enthusiastic practitioner. We have no way of knowing whether we have succeeded. We also set out to provide material that would help you:

(a) develop insight into your own interpersonal skills so that you might be better able to use them effectively and to overcome barriers that you may meet;

(b) learn specialist skills, should you wish to, and/or extend your skills to specialist settings;

(c) identify and use particular strategies in particular situations, and to handle the effects of the strategies you chose;

(d) explore the constraints that limit your effective use of interpersonal skills in various settings.

We think we have supplied the material, but again have no way of knowing whether it has worked for you.

Throughout, we have tried to go beyond the simple behaviours that are essential parts of any interpersonal skill, to include cognitive and contextual aspects. We would like to emphasize that interpersonal skill is not just what you do: it is also the ability to reflect on why you do what you do, and what effect on both yourself and other people your actions have. All the time, though, interpersonal behaviours both create and arise from specific interaction contexts. So we would wish to stress the point we made in the Introduction, that interpersonal skill is a process and not an end point, and as such is never finally achieved. We all have a responsibility to ourselves and the other people we are involved with, to keep monitoring our interpersonal effectiveness, and it is this willingness and ability to keep reflecting openly about ourselves that is, arguably, the most vital part of interpersonal skill.

Reflections on material that is excluded

There are some crucial areas of interpersonal skills for nurses that we have not touched upon, and the book would be incomplete if we made no mention of them.

Most of the discussion and examples have been of nurse–patient/relative interaction, and yet a great deal of our relationships are with colleagues. A full discussion of interpersonal skills for nurses should include encounters with other nurses and people from other professions or occupations. It is as important for hospital patients to witness good-quality interaction between staff as it is for them to receive it. We would urge you, when considering staff relationships, to explore the possibilities for promoting cooperation between staff: there is an overwhelming tendency for us to concentrate on handling conflict!

In a similar vein, we are conscious that very few examples have been drawn from community settings. We apologize for this, and hope that those of you who work in the community settings can extend the ideas we have presented in a way that makes them fit your experiences. We would say again, though, that we do not believe interpersonal skills can just be learnt once and for all, and transported into any setting. The constraints that operate in the community will vary, and if we take note of the notion that interpersonal skills both create and arise from specific interaction contexts, the skills themselves may also vary.

Although many of the exercises we suggested required you to discuss the issues in small groups, we have not included group interaction skills *per se*. We do not think it is enough to take your repertoire of interpersonal skills into a group setting, and expect to be fully effective (although it is a necessary start!). Group interaction skills require a lot more in the way of understanding

— and experiencing — the dynamics of different kinds of groups. If you do have a lot of group interactions, as most of us find we do if we stop to think about it, and would like to explore group skills some more, we urge you to attend some basic courses in group work, or at the very least explore some of the experiential literature (see Appendix III).

Throughout the book we have restricted our discussions to common nursing situations that are (we think) morally uncontentious. There is a range of skills, though, that some of you may find you need to use more and more as contraction in the health care services continues. After a while you may feel that patient well-being has been subordinated to political will and organizational convenience to such an extent that you must take a stand. By then, the interpersonal skills of protest, confrontation, negotiation and patient advocacy may be the ones you will need. These are not the skills commonly found in a compendium of interpersonal skills for nurses.

Future directions

There is no doubt that interest in interpersonal aspects of nursing is growing. If we are correct in our assertions that interpersonal skills both create and arise from the interaction context, training individual nurses to acquire the skills may not result in dramatic increases in the quality of patient care. Assuming that the best conditions for nurses to learn interpersonal skills are created, we still cannot guarantee that they will be able to use them. At the same time as support for the development and use of interpersonal skills is being offered by the nursing profession, the delivery of health care services is being judged by very different criteria, namely time efficiency and value for money as manifest in performance indicators and cost limits, for example. We in the field of interpersonal skill must continually protest that such criteria necessarily exclude any consideration of the quality of interpersonal relationships, and thereby the quality of total patient care. Thus, increasingly, interpersonal skills in nursing are becoming a political issue.

TUTOR NOTES FOR THE EXERCISES

We have included some tutor notes to accompany the exercises. These notes are meant to be guidelines for those who have done little in the way of either experiential teaching, or communications/interpersonal skills teaching before. They have been written in a way that adapts the exercises in the text from ones that individual students can follow, to class activities. For the necessary instructions and the accompanying answer sheets tutors are referred back to the given exercise in the main part of the text. The exercises are not meant to be prescriptive, and are only intended to give some hints of how to manage class sessions. We hope they are useful, but do urge tutors to be flexible in their use. No two teaching situations are the same, and the exercises will be most effective if tutors can modify them to suit their own conditions. We have offered some suggestions for materials to use in the exercises. Certainly, we would consider some basic stock of materials to be essential for interpersonal skills teaching. Specifically, we would recommend that tutors have available blackboard and chalk; overhead projector; large (poster size–A1) sheets of paper; plenty of felt markers; blue tac or similar; tape recorders and a good supply of paper and pencils. Some of the exercises need additional 'props', and these are mentioned if relevant.

The exercises vary in their format, but basically are variations of structured small group exercises. The sizes of the small groups vary from pairs to groups of eight (groups larger than 6–8 mean that they are unlikely to encourage full participation from all the members). Some exercises include work in the large class group. The format for particular exercises can vary: we have given examples of ways of working that we have found successful. Please experiment!

It may be useful to bear in mind some principles of good practice for using structured exercises such as those we have included here.

(a) Be well prepared. Try to anticipate the unexpected as well as the predictable.

(b) Vary the format of each session. Keep student interest up by varying the activities in a particular session as well as those between sessions.

(c) Always take care to leave enough time to process the work that students have been engaged in (approximately five times the length of the exercise). Encourage students to feel their views and experiences are valuable.

(d) If students give any feedback about the way the sessions are being run, take note of any suggestions they make.

(e) Try to ensure that sessions are enjoyable — this is the best way to ensure the 'lessons learnt' will stay with the students when they enter the reality of clinical nursing, where interpersonal issues are not always (usually!) given much prominence.

Chapter 2

Exercise 2.1 Explorations of personal identity

Time

1 hour or homework

Preparation

1. Instructions and answer sheets for every student.
2. Large sheets of paper, felt markers, blue tac or similar.

Organization

1. Issue instructions and answer sheets, and ask students to complete the first three sections individually.
2. Combine to groups of four. Ask groups to prepare definitions of 'self' and 'personality' based on their replies to the proceding sections, and in the

light of the discussion issues. Ask each group to write their definitions on large sheets of paper to display to the rest of the class.

3. Display the posters around the room and invite students to look at them all.

4. When all the students have seen the posters, hold general discussion highlighting similarities and differences between the definitions. Explore any issues arising from the discussion issues.

Note

It is unlikely that everyone will be able to think of 20 replies to the question 'Who am I?' After they have been working at their replies for about 8 minutes, tell the class that they should simply think of as many replies as they can, and not to worry if they cannot think of 20. Some students may look up the definitions in the dictionary — if they do, ask them to compile their own definitions as well, and to compare them with the dictionary ones.

Exercise 2.2 Life histories: positive selves

Time

1 hour (depending on the size of the class)

Preparation

1. Instructions for all students.
2. Large (poster-size) sheets of paper, felt markers and blue tac or similar.

Organization

1. Issue instructions and ask all students to work individually on the 'story of their lives', with a view to displaying the posters and talking about them.

2. After 20 minutes, either display the posters around the room and invite all students to view them, asking 'artists' for clarification as required, *or* ask each student to talk through her/his poster to a group of six colleagues. No student should be expected to answer questions she/he does not wish to.

3. Reconvene the large group and consider the discussion issues. Briefly summarize the discussion on the board.

Note

This exercise can raise emotional memories. It is essential that the objectives of looking at positive strengths is adhered to. Some students may be at a loss for how to draw their pictures. If they are, suggest they draw a 'life snake' (see below). It is essential that enough time is given at the end of the session for students to 'wind down'. Tutor should be prepared to draw her/his own 'life story' if asked to do so.

Life snake

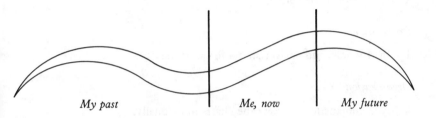

My past   Me, now   My future

Exercise 2.3 Personal values and self-esteem

Time

45 minutes

Preparation

1.   Instructions and answer sheets for all students.

Organization

1.   Ask students to complete charts individually.
2.   Ask students to join with a partner with whom to discuss their valued characteristics in the light of the discussion issues.
3.   Reconvene the large group and discuss (briefly) the notion that values are central to our being and are difficult to change, producing traumatic effects if ever they do change. Conclude in terms of self-awareness being a process that contributes to raised self-esteem.

Note

Some students may find it hard to think of the characteristics they do/do not admire. It is a good idea to have a list of characteristics to give to students: they can then rate their chosen people and themselves on them.

Exercise 2.4 Beliefs about nursing

Time

20 minutes or homework

Preparations

1. Instructions and answer sheets for all students.

Organization

1. Ask students to complete the charts individually.
2. Reconvene the large group and ask for examples of each type of belief. Draw up a list of the different types of beliefs about nursing on the board/flipchart/overhead projector.
3. Briefly consider the discussion issues and conclude by examining the differences between values and beliefs.

Note

There should be no problems conducting this exercise. If some types of beliefs are difficult for students to identify, use this as the basis for discussion and as a possible criticism of this method of classifying beliefs.

Exercise 2.5 Self-perception and feedback from others

Time

1 hour

Preparation

1. Instructions for every group of eight.

Organization

. Divide the class into groups of 6–8 and issue instructions for the game. Talk the class through the instructions and answer any queries.
. After 30 minutes, call the game to a halt and ask the groups to consider their experiences in the light of the discussion issues. Circulate around the groups and ensure that discussion is constructive.
. Reconvene the large group and summarize the class experience. Conclude by drawing attention to the fact that other people generally see us differently from the ways we perceive ourselves.

Note

This exercise can be embarrassing for the 'underchosen' and 'overchosen' members. Tutor should endeavour to ensure that the number of choices is raised constructively in the discussion.

Participants may try and play 'safe' by always choosing, for example, physical characteristics that are obvious (such as 'tallest', 'wearing red', and so on). If this happens, tutor could suggest they play a round mentioning only *internal* characteristics.

Care should be taken to ensure that enough time is devoted to processing the game, and that nobody leaves feeling uncomfortable. It is usually quite easy to direct the discussion constructively around the issues involved in self-presentation: if group members know each other well, the discussion may lead to conflict between people. The conflict should be dealt with in the group, or privately afterwards with the people concerned.

Exercise 2.6 Perception of known and unknown others

Time

45 minutes

Preparation

1. Plenty of pictures of (a) unknown and (b) well-known (preferably controversial) people, for example, from newspapers, magazines, etc. The pictures could be presented on slides if resources permit.
2. Instructions and answer sheets for all students.

Organization

1. Divide the class into groups of four. Ask each group to look at eac
   picture presented and to discuss the answers to the questions on th
   charts.
2. Combine to groups of eight and consider the discussion issues.
3. Ask each group to compile a list of the cues used to make judgemen
   about known and unknown people.
4. Reconvene the large group and draw up a composite list of cues used
   make judgements about known and unknown people. Display list o
   board/flipchart/overhead projector.
5. Conclude session by raising the issue of the role that cues with person
   relevance play in our perceptions of others.

Note

There should be no problems conducting this exercise.

Exercise 2.7 Self as 'agent' and lack of control

Time

Homework followed by 30-minute discussion.

Preparation

Instructions and answer sheets for every student.

Organization

1. Issue instructions for students to complete exercise as homework. Set
   date for the follow-up session and ask students to bring their complete
   charts to it.
2. *Follow-up* ask students to describe one of their incidents to the rest of th
   class. Select students at random and choose equal numbers of the tw
   types of situation. If numbers permit, ensure that everyone has a chanc
   to describe one incident.
3. As the situations are described, ask people to consider the discussio
   issues.
4. Conclude with a general discussion about the cultural context of lack o
   control and its contribution to low self-esteem, possibly lack of self
   confidence.

Note

Some students may not have done their homework. Do not make an issue of this. However, if several have not done it, it may be worth exploring reasons for this in the large group. Discuss student responsibility for doing work and for contributing to group discussions. This may raise some animosity to the teaching methods and/or content of the course. These should be dealt with in the group if they are shared or privately if they are expressed by only one or two students. Do not ignore these feelings.

Chapter 3

Exercise 3.1 Taxonomy of non-verbal behaviour

Time

30 minutes

Preparation

Instructions and answer sheets for all students.

Organization

1. Divide the class into pairs or into groups of three (including O — observer) and issue instructions and answer sheets.
2. After 25 minutes, join groups to form groups of six and ask students to consider the discussion issues.
3. After 10 minutes, either hear the groups' lists of non-verbal behaviours and compile a composite list on the board, or present a chart of the taxonomy of non-verbal behaviours (see Table 3.1 for example). Explain any element that may not have been mentioned by the students. Raise the possibility that different behaviours would have been emitted by (a) older people, and (b) people from different cultural backgrounds, and conclude.

Note

There should be no problems conducting this exercise.

Exercise 3.2 Habits and change

Time

45 minutes

Preparation

Instructions for every student.

Organization

1. Divide the class into groups of three and issue instructions. Read the instructions to the class and clarify any queries.
2. Combine groups to form groups of six to consider the discussion issues.
3. Ask each group to report on what had happened to the conversations during the exercise. Draw out the implications of the difficulty of changing habits for the learning and development of interpersonal skills. Emphasize the importance of practice. Consider some examples from the nursing field, of situations where interaction is hindered by one of the parties trying to behave 'unnaturally'.

Note

The two people talking may need to be reminded to think carefully about those behaviours they are trying to change. O may need to be prompted to remind A and B! In the classroom, the conversations should be allowed to continue until the speakers 'dry up'. It is just possible that there is little disruption of the conversation, although this is unlikely. In such circumstances, ask students to think about any situation where their self-consciousness has led them to interact in a strange manner. Ask the students for ideas of how they think the issues could be illustrated in the classroom, and take heed!

Exercise 3.3 Encounter regulation

Time

20 minutes

Preparation

1. Instructions for every student.
2. Enough blindfolds for half the class.

Organization

1. Divide the class into pairs and issue the instructions.
2. After both conversations have been held, and notes been written, combine pairs to groups of six and invite students to share their experiences in the light of the discussion issues.
3. Ask a representative of each group to relate the substance of the group discussion. Produce a summary of (a) the nursing situations that were identified and (b) the strategies that could be used to balance the interaction on the board. Students should be encouraged to take a copy of the summary.
4. Conclude with short summary of the role of non-verbal behaviours in the 'meshing' of ordinary conversations and the regulation of encounters. If necessary, illustrate with the example of interaction breakdown in telephone conversations.

Note

Some students may giggle. Give them a chance to recover, but if this is impossible call the exercise to a halt. Hold a general discussion of nursing situations wherein one person has far fewer cues to the other person's non-verbal behaviour. Consider what would (or does) happen in such circumstances and how nurses can help to overcome any feelings of discomfort. Ask the students for any ideas of how these points could best be illustrated in the classroom and take heed!

Exercise 3.4 Rules of conversations

Time

1 hour

Preparation

1. Lists of conversations.
2. Cards with the title of one conversation written on each.

3. Large sheets of paper, felt markers and blue tac or similar.
4. Discussion issues for distribution.

Organization

1. Divide class into groups of four. Give each group a different conversation to consider, ask the groups to write the 'rules for the conversation' they have received.
2. Ask each group to list the rules on a large sheet of paper to be displayed to the class.
3. Ask each group to consider the same conversation and to list the rules that would apply if it were taking place between partners with an age difference of twenty years, and to list these rules on a separate sheet of paper, making it clear which partner is the younger one.
4. Ask groups to display their lists of rules, making sure that the conversation title is not included.
5. Distribute the whole list of conversations to the class, and ask students to identify which set of rules represents which of the conversations.
6. Combine groups to groups of eight to check answers and to consider the discussion issues.
7. As a large group, hear (briefly) what each smaller group had discussed. Conclude by exploring the consequences for interactions when the rules of conversation are broken.

Note

There should be no problems conducting this exercise as long as students are clear as to what 'rules of conversation' mean.

Exercise 3.5 Instruction and attenuated communication

Time

45 minutes

Preparation

1. Sets of three rectangular pieces of paper for each person (approximately 20 cm × 10 cm).
2. Instructions and discussion issues for every student.

Organization

1. Divide class into pairs and issue sets of paper. Ask students to carry out the task as indicated on the instructions.
2. After pairs have discussed the reasons for disparities in their arrangements, reconvene the class and consider the discussion issues.
3. Conclude with some comments about the value of questions for:

   (a) clarification,
   (b) checking that a person has understood or followed instructions correctly,
   (c) asking a person how an explanation might be made more clear,
   (d) encouraging elaborated code when necessary.

Note

Students may present too easy a pattern to their partners. If this happens, suggest that they start off with as difficult an arrangement as possible. It can sometimes be necessary for the tutor to arrange the papers irregularly for a particular pair, and then to proceed as above. If the pattern is too easy, the discussion will be uninteresting and the exercise may seem to be pointless.

Exercise 3.6 Language codes

Time

Homework followed by 1 hour.

Preparation

Instructions for all students.

Organization

1. Issue all students with the homework instructions and tell them when the follow-up session will be. Ask them to bring the samples of their conversations to the follow-up session.
2. *Follow-up:* Combine to groups of four. Ask students to listen to each other's conversations and consider the discussion issues in relation to them.

3. Reconvene the large group. Ask representatives of each of the small groups to give examples from their conversations of different discussion issues. Ask all groups for the essence of their replies to the last question.
4. Give a brief résumé of the interdependence of verbal and non-verbal behaviours. Emphasize that a lot of reactions (especially emotional reactions) to what is said are because of the non-verbal cues accompanying the speech.
5. Conclude with a brief discussion of the amount of material that must have been lost due to memory (or lack of it). Note that the only accurate way to record speech is via audio/video tape recordings, but to do this involves ethical issues that are perhaps greater than those involved in just 'listening in' to a conversation. Consider whether or not there were any ethical issues involved in conducting this exercise. Did anyone tell the people she/he had listened to, how she/he was going to use the conversation? Why/why not?

Note

The whole of this exercise can be done as homework.

Some students may not have collected a conversation, or may have felt unable to eavesdrop or to remember it sufficiently to write it down. If only a few students have been unable to do it, try to ensure that they are evenly spread among the discussion groups. If a lot of students have failed to bring a conversation, it may be worth spending some time discussing why this is and to consider the problems they had.

Whatever the reason for failing to bring a conversation to the session, all students should be encouraged to explore the discussion issues. It is a good idea to bring some 'reserve' conversations to the session. If you do not have time to prepare your own samples, use some of those that are available from the nursing press, or from commercial packages (see Appendix III). Check copyright regulations before mass-producing such material.

Exercise 3.7 Functions and strategies of speech (1)

Time

Homework, followed by 15-minute session.

Preparation

1. Copies of Table 3.2 for all students.
2. Instructions for all students.

Organization

1. Issue homework instructions and tell students the date for the follow-up session.
2. During the follow-up session, ask students whether any of them had found it hard to think of examples for any particular functions. Allow the class to provide examples of such strategies.
3. Conclude by checking that all students understand Table 3.2.

Note

Some students may not have completed their homework. If this happens, remind students that homework and completion of exercises are an essential part of their learning, and that only they can take responsibility for this. It is a good idea to have some ready examples of strategies representing all the functions in case there are some that the class cannot supply.

Exercise 3.8 Functions and strategies of speech (2)

Time

As long as is available.

Preparation

1. Video tapes of nursing interactions that have good-quality sound tracks. Commercial ones are available (see Appendix III). If it is difficult to obtain these, video tapes of any social behaviour would suffice. Failing this, issue samples of conversations such as those featured in the Talking Points series (*Nursing Times*, 1982). Check copyright regulations before mass-producing such material.
2. Instructions and answer sheets for all students.

Organization

1. Show a nursing interaction on video tape/issue a nursing conversation for students to read. Ask students to note down any observations they have about the encounter on their observation chart.
2. Repeat for another interaction, and so on for as many interactions as possible, whilst maintaining student interest.
3. In either small groups (4–6) or as a class, consider the discussion issues. Summarize the major issues on the board.
4. Conclude by reiterating the points raised in the discussion, emphasizing the notion that effective interpersonal skills are judged by their effect (i.e. what happens afterwards) and therefore *perceptual* skills are just as important as *performance* skills if we are to adjust our behaviour.

Note

This exercise is time consuming as it stimulates a lot of discussion. At this stage, it may be useful to limit the discussion to the discussion issues: as students get more experienced at recognizing the effects of interpersonal skills, and better able to give informed (rather than impressionistic) ideas of how the sequences could have been enacted more appropriately, the exercise can be repeated.

Exercise 3.9 Observation of social behaviour

Time

Homework with 30-minute follow-up (this exercise could be used as a written assignment).

Preparation

Instructions for all students.

Organization

1. Issue students with instructions and tell them when the follow-up session will be.
2. Follow-up session: Divide the class into groups of four and ask students to share their observations, and to consider the discussion issues. Ask each

group to prepare a summary of the group members' experiences to feedback to the large group.

3. Hear each group's summary. Summarize the points to emerge under the following headings:

   (a) Problems of observing social behaviour; non-verbal and speech.
   (b) Criteria used in the interpretation of social behaviour.
   (c) The influence of 'self' on the interpretation of social behaviour.

4. Conclude the session by reiterating the value of considering both verbal and non-verbal elements of social behaviour: emphasize their interdependence in the attribution of meaning.

   Draw attention to the influence of the setting (sub)culture and the 'self' on the interpretation of social behaviour, and stress the notion that 'correct' observation and interpretation is virtually impossible without extensive training, but that sensitivity to the issues is the first step towards being able to make effective use of interpersonal skills.

Note

It is likely that students will have noted more non-verbal than verbal behaviours. This may be because they were reluctant to get close enough to their 'targets' to hear what they were saying. If this is so, consider whether they can make any sensible interpretation of what is going on, and whether misunderstandings arise in nursing contexts due to a similar lack of the full information.

If this exercise is used as a written assignment, it may be necessary to give students some ideas as to what is expected of them in terms of incorporating the issues raised throughout Chapter 3.

Exercise 3.10 Expectations and labelling

Time

Homework with brief follow-up session in next interpersonal skills class

Preparation

Instructions and answer sheets for all students.

Organization

1. Issue instructions and set follow-up date.
2. *Follow-up*: Check whether students had any problems with the exercise.
3. Conclude by emphasizing that the exercise is designed to help students clarify *labelling* as distinct from other role expectations. Hold brief discussion on the basis of students' answers to the questions in the exercise and to the discussion issues.

Note

This exercise requires little processing. As with all structured exercises, time should be given for any students to raise matters of interest of personal concern that have arisen from the exercise.

Exercise 3.11 Stereotyping

Time

40 minutes

Preparation

1. Prepare three sets of stereotype labels (13 cm × 7 cm index cards are useful):

    (a) Everyone in the class has had some experience of, for example, staff canteen food, nurse tutors, student nurses, friends, etc.
    (b) Class may have had some information about, for example, intensive therapy units, gynaecologists, physiotherapists etc.
    (c) Class may have heard about for example, good patients, schizophrenics, sheltered housing, etc.
2. Discussion issues to distribute.

Organization

1. Split the class into groups of four. Distribute stereotype label cards between the groups, ensuring that each group gets at least one from each set.
2. Issue the following instructions to the groups: Please think about the label your group has been given. Working individually, describe what you think the typical characteristics associated with that label are. Use any

information you can, including your past experience. You have 5 minutes. You will not have to read your list out, but will be expected to discuss it with your group. Any questions?

3. Clarify any questions. After 5 minutes ask the students to share their answers with the other members of the group. Ask groups to elect a spokesperson to prepare a summary of the discussion in relation to the discussion issues.

4. Hear each group's summary and present the major points on the board under the different stereotype lables. Draw attention to differences between labels that all group members (a) have direct experience of, (b) have some information about, (c) may have heard about. Point out that the process of stereotyping according to role is similar to that of labelling.

Note

There should be no problems in conducting this exercise.

Exercise 3.12 Implicit personality theories

Time

30–40 minutes.

Preparation

1. Instructions and answer sheets for each student.
2. Large sheets of paper and sets of felt markers for each group of three, blue tac or similar.

Organization

1. Ask each student to complete the answer sheet *working individually*. Stress that they will not be required to read out their answers, but will be expected to share them with others.
2. Combine to groups of three and compare answers. Consider the discussion issues.
3. Ask each group to prepare a summary poster of (a) sources of the judgements made and (b) examples of implicit personality theories that have been used in members' nursing career so far.

4. Display the posters and invite students to look at them. Allow sufficient time for the class to examine all the posters. Conclude session by stressing that we all do (and will) use implicit personality theories, and that they are a useful way of handling information about people. We should, though, be aware that they may be incorrect!

Note

Tutor/students may be embarrassed doing this exercise with tutor as 'target'. A variation would be for students, in threes, to describe a fourth person known to them all. Proceed as before.

Exercise 3.13 Central traits and consistency

Time

Homework with 30 minutes follow-up session.

Preparation

Instructions and answer sheets for every student.

Organization

1. Ask students to complete the answer sheet and bring them to the next session. Give date of follow-up session.
2. In the follow-up session ask students to combine in groups of four and discuss their answers. Ask them to pay particular attention to their views on the question 'How might the issue of "consistency around central traits" affect your interpersonal behaviour as a nurse?'
3. Hold a general discussion with examples from the groups of how behaviour as a nurse may be affected by the 'consistency around central traits' issue.

Note

As with all the homework tasks there may be a problem of students failing to complete it. Stress the importance of doing the homework for the follow-up session.

Exercise 3.14 Selective perception

Time

3 minutes followed by 20 minutes later in session.

Preparation

1. Arrange for a confederate unknown to the class to interrupt the session. Have details of the characteristics of the confederate with reference to the answer sheet.
2. Instructions and answer sheets for every student.

Organization

1. During a lecture/discussion, arrange for the confederate to interrupt the session. Ensure that there is some interaction, so that the attention of the class is brought to the interruption. Comment on the interruption in passing with humour/impatience etc.
2. Later in the session issue students with the answer sheets and ask them to complete them individually.
3. Combine in groups of three or four and compare answers. Consider the discussion issues.
4. After about 15 minutes reconvene the large group and describe the person accurately. Discuss the implications of selective perception for nursing.

Note

There is no reason why this exercise should not take place during the 'lecture' component on social perception. Students are unlikely to suspect anything. To draw their attention to the interruption, it may be necessary to comment quite a bit on the person (for example, 'She's always doing this/she is funny — a senior tutor, and always forgetting the chalk, etc.'). Some students may be embarrassed/annoyed at the deception involved. Ensure that feelings of this sort are recognized and defused.

Exercise 3.15 Reconstruction of memory

Time

40 minutes

Preparation

1. Messages written on separate cards (see page 332).
2. Tape recorders to record the progress of the message — optional.
3. Discussion issues to distribute.

Organization

1. Split the class into groups of between 6 and 15. Ask the members to number themselves.
2. Ask the first person in each group to receive a different message from the tutor and to stand away from the group. One by one the members of the group are asked to receive the message from the person before them. Successive deliveries of the message can be recorded.
3. The last person in the group is asked to write down the message.
4. Reconvene the large group. If tape recorders were used ask each group to play the sequence of messages. If no tape recorders were used, hear the first and last versions of each group's message.
5. As a large group, consider the discussion issues with tutor summarizing main points on the board.

Note

This exercise can be funny and enjoyment should be encouraged. Students may want to do 'repeat' messages, so plan for repetition — have plenty of sample messages. It may be useful to have some of the recommendations offered in Section 3.4 on giving information to hand. Take care that members of the group do not overhear the message before it is their turn. If tape recorders are used ensure that each speaker is far enough from other speakers for an adequate recording to be made.

Chapter 4

Exercise 4.1 Role strain

Time

Homework followed by 15-minute session.

Preparation

1. Instructions and answer sheets for every student.
2. Copies of Figure 4.1 for each person.

Organization

1. Ask each student to complete the diagrams illustrating different sources of role strain as shown on the answer sheets. Set date for follow-up session.
2. In follow-up session, as a large group, consider the discussion issues.
3. Terminate discussion by referring to the notion that 'self' can be considered a role, and as such is defined by others. What implications does a role analysis have for understanding popular and unpopular patients?

Note

Students may find it difficult completing some of the diagrams. Tutor should have some further examples to show on overhead projector, to illustrate fully the approach.

Exercise 4.2 Group identification

Time

30–45 minutes

Preparation

1. Sheets of newspaper or any typewritten passage for every student.
2. Discussion issues to distribute or present on overhead projector.

Organization

1. Issue each student with a fairly long typewritten passage.
2. Read out the following instructions: This is a task that I want you to do now: we will consider the results in a later session. It's a task concerned with the recognition of letters. I'd like you to start at the *end* of the passage. Read backwards and cross off every letter that has an angle in it (for example, *k, v, w, y,* etc.). I want you to do this for one minute. Do you understand? Wait for any questions and clarify the task.) O.K., start now.

3. After 1 minute stop the activity. Ask students to count the number of letters crossed off and to call out their totals. Write the totals on the board looking increasingly puzzled as more accumulate. Add them up and find the average number crossed off.

4. Look very concerned at the average and say, 'That's really a very low number of letters to have found. Last year's students got, on average (cite a number 10–15 more than the present average). Look, do it again and we'll see what it comes to. Mark where you got to last time and just carry on. I'll give you a minute again. O.K.? Right, start now.'

5. After a minute call a stop, and ask for the totals to be called out again. Write them on the board. It may not be necessary to find the average as the totals will probably be considerably higher than the first time.

6. Assuming the totals (and average) have gone up, as a large group consider the discussion issues.

7. Conclude discussion by noting that the effect could be produced by practice — but it is unlikely. Similarly, there is no knowledge whether the totals *really* increased, or whether the number of errors increased and/or just the report of totals increased. Suggest that an important influence was the group identification influence. Some individuals may not have increased their totals overall, but the group did, though. So group identification processes operate differently for different people. Apologize for the deception involved.

Note

It is just possible that the total does not increase. In this case tell the group that it usually does and have the discussion on the basis of what *usually* happens. Consider why it did not happen in this case.

Exercise 4.3 Interaction openings

Time

30 minutes (plus homework — optional)

Preparation

1. Enough answer sheets for every student.
2. Copies of Table 4.1 for every student.

Organization

1. Ask students to consider appropriate interaction openings and complete the answer sheets in pairs.
2. Combine in groups of six and compare examples.
3. Critically appraise the examples with reference to the discussion issues. Ask each group to select the best examples of each opening to present to the whole group.
4. As a large group hear each small group's best examples. Consider the functions they serve. Have some functions not been covered? Why?
5. Conclude by stressing the ritualistic nature of interaction openings and by noting that ritual may obscure individual expression/needs.

Note

There should be no problems with this exercise. It is a good idea to have some model examples (both 'good' and 'bad') just in case the small group discussion is limited. This exercise can be done as a *role play* exercise. Use groups of 4–6, with two 'players' (changing for each of the examples) and the rest being observers who note down features of the interaction openings for critical appraisal.

Homework (optional)

Ask students to collect some examples of interaction openings. In a follow-up session consider whether or not they were effective. Why were they effective/ineffective? What functions did they serve?

Exercise 4.4 Interaction closures

Time

30 minutes (plus homework — optional)

Preparation

1. Enough answer sheets for every student.
2. Copies of Table 4.2 for every student.

Organization

1. Ask students to consider appropriate interaction closures and to complete the answer sheets in pairs.
2. Combine to groups of six and compare examples.
3. Critically appraise the examples with reference to the discussion issues. Ask each group to select the best examples of each closure to present to the whole group.
4. As a large group, hear each small group's best example. Consider the functions they serve. Have some functions not been covered? Why?
5. Conclude by stressing the ritualistic nature of interaction closures and by noting that ritual may obscure individual expression/needs.

Note

There should be no problems with this exercise. It is a good idea to have some model examples (both 'good' and 'bad') just in case the small group discussion is limited. This exercise can be done as a role play exercise. Use groups of 4–6, with two 'players' (changing for each of the examples), and the rest being observers who note down features of the interaction closures for critical appraisal.

Homework (optional)

Ask students to collect some examples of interaction closures. In a follow-up session consider whether or not they were effective. Why were they effective/ineffective? What functions did they serve?

Chapter 5

Exercise 5.1 The interpretation of facial and vocal cues of emotion

Time

15 minutes

Preparation

1. Instructions and answer sheets for every student.
2. Completed chart to distribute or present on an overhead projector.

Organization

1. Ask each student to complete chart, working individually.
2. In pairs, ask students to discuss their answers, paying particular attention to any disagreements.
3. Present completed chart.
4. Combine in groups of six to consider discussion issues. Each group to prepare a summary.
5. Very briefly, as a large group, hear each group's summary. Summarize the points on the board, without holding extensive further discussion, and conclude.

Note

There should be no problems in conducting this exercise.

Exercise 5.2 The expression and recognition of emotion

Time

40 minutes

Preparation

1. Instructions and answer sheets for every student.
2. Sets of questions (see page 334) for B in second part of exercise.

Organization

I. *Non-verbal expression*
1. Ask pairs of students to follow the instructions and to complete the answer sheets.

II. *Contradictory messages*
2. In pairs, ask student to read the instructions and to complete the answer sheets. *Issue B with the sets of sentences on page 333–4.*

3. Combine in groups of six to consider discussion issues. Ask each group to prepare a summary.
4. Very briefly, as a large group, hear each group's summary. Summarize the points on the board, and without holding extensive further discussion, conclude.

Note

Students may giggle, especially with the counting and contradictory messages tasks. It is probably a good idea to say that you know they are likely to giggle when you introduce the exercise. Tell the students that it does not matter if they giggle a bit, as long as they recover sufficiently to carry out the task.

If students do giggle, and this gets out of hand, either hold a general discussion as to why this type of task should make them giggle (embarrassment, revealing their own shortcomings, etc.) or move straight on to the discussion groups. At the end of the session, ask the students if they can think of any ways that the points could have been illustrated without reducing them to giggles: if they come up with any suggestions, take heed!

Exercise 5.3 Display rules and the expression of emotions

Time

30–40 minutes

Preparation

1. Instructions and answer sheets for every student.

Organization

1. Split class into groups of four. Allocate each group a different role from the nursing context (for example, nurse, patient, ward sister, doctor, relative, child, etc.) Ask each group to complete the chart with respect to their allocated role.
2. Combine in groups of eight and consider the discussion issues. Ask each group to prepare a summary.

3. Very briefly, as a large group, hear each group's summary. Summarize the points on the board without holding extensive further discussion and conclude by drawing attention to the importance of context and 'display rules' for the understanding of emotion.

Note

Students may need some prompting to think of different circumstances where an emotion may be inappropriate. It may be a good idea to have some examples in mind for each of the different roles before the start, and to float between groups during the discussions.

Exercise 5.4 Interpretation of interpersonal attitudes

Time

30–45 minutes

Preparation

1. Instructions and charts for every student.
2. Pictures to distribute *or* slides to show *or* sections of video tapes (for example Communication in Patient Care Tapes, see Appendix III) depicting nurses at work, illustrating at the most *10* different attitudes to other people. (If video tapes are being used, allow more time.)

Organization

1. Issue each student with a set of pictures, *or* show the slides one at a time, *or* show a short section of video tape at a time.
2. Ask each student to complete the chart with respect to each of the target pictures.
3. In groups of six, compare answers and discuss the reasons for any disagreements. Allow any group that wishes to see any of the target pictures again, to do so.
4. Combine to large group and consider the discussion issues.
5. Summarize points on the board as they arise in discussion, and conclude with reference to the importance of context for the understanding of interpersonal attitudes.

Note

In the large group, a few students may dominate the group. Do not draw attention to this and attempt to embarrass those that speak a lot, nor attempt to shame others into more involvement. If some students are disruptive in their participation, point out that one of the ways we achieve dominance (as an interpersonal attitude) is by talking a lot!

Exercise 5.5 Listening

Time

45 minutes

Preparation

Sets of instructions for groups of three.

Organization

1. In groups of three, allocate the roles of A (speaker), B (listener) and O (observer). Issue sets of instructions.
2. After all three conversations have been held, combine in a large group. Ask each small group for an example of how any one of their B's could have been a 'better' listener. Integrate in terms of the requirements for effective listening (see Section 5.4). In the large group consider the discussion issues.
3. Summarize points on the board and conclude in terms of the relationship between effective listening and reward in interaction.

Note

Students may find it difficult to think of conversations. O's may sometimes be poor at recording what B is doing, or of thinking how she/he could be a 'better' listener. It is a good idea to 'float' between groups to help them record behaviour, if necessary.

Exercise 5.6 Touch

Time

30 minutes

Preparation

1. Instructions and charts for every student.
2. Prepare several front-back pairs (six is a manageable number) with different labels on them. Choose labels that are linked with some other aspects of students' training (for example, that relate to their clinical practice).

Organization

1. Ask each student to shade the figure.
2. Issue all students with either identical or different labels to the figures.
3. Ask each student to shade the figures according to the instructions.
4. Combine in pairs to discuss the shading, paying particular attention to any disagreements.
5. Combine in groups of six. Ask each group to choose the five most important points, in order of priority, relating to the use of touch in nursing. Ask each group to consider the discussion issues and to prepare a summary.
6. As a large group, collate a list of the issues raised by the small groups on the board. Conclude with reference to the distinction between touch in the execution of a nursing task, and touch with a social meaning. Can the two functions be distinguished?

Note

There may be some giggling. It is a good idea to say, when the exercise is introduced, that you will be expecting some giggling. If it persists, either go straight to the discussion groups or hold some discussion about the embarrassing nature of 'touch' and whether there are cultural differences in the extent of the embarrassment it causes. If giggling occurs in the small groups, go to the group and try to turn it into a constructive issue by, for example, asking students if there have been any occasions in their nursing careers where they have been embarrassed by something to do with touching patients.

Exercise 5.7 Self-disclosure

Time

30 minutes

Preparation

Instructions and charts for every student.

Organization

1. Ask each student to complete the charts, and then to combine to groups of four to share their answers and consider the discussion issues.
2. Ask each group to prepare a summary.
3. Very briefly, as a large group, hear the small groups' summaries. Write the major points on the board without holding extensive further discussion. Conclude in terms of the importance of the situation for choosing appropriate self-disclosures.

Note

Students may find it embarrassing to discuss self-disclosure. If they do, draw the discussion round to cultural differences in the sanctioning of self-disclosure. If it is pointed out that even though the chart has a category of 'intimate' disclosures, this is more usefully seen as a dimension, and there will always be more intimate disclosures possible, student anxieties about revealing 'intimate secrets' should decrease.

Chapter 6

Exercise 6.1 Speech elicitation

Time

30–40 minutes

Preparation

1. Instructions and discussion issues for every student. Make sure you have instructions for person B as well (see page 334).
2. Large sheets of paper, felt markers and blue tac or similar.

Organization

1. Split the class into pairs, A and B (or threes, A, B and O — observer).
2. Ask all the As to leave the room, walk down the corridor/stairs and then to return.
3. While As are out of the room, instruct Bs (see page 334).
4. Observers — take notes on the interaction between A and B as fully as possible. Try to resist giving any further clarification in response to queries from B.
5. As soon as possible, invite As back into the room and invite them to talk to their partners.
6. After about 10 minutes, or as soon as most of the pairs have dried up, call a stop to the task. Allow a few minutes for B to explain the instructions she/he had been given, and the pairs to discuss the exercise as a whole.
7. Combine to groups of six and discuss the exercise with reference to the discussion issues. Ask each group to summarize the strategies that B used to encourage A to elaborate, on large sheets of paper which are to be posted around the room.
8. Display the posters, and invite the students to look at all of the summaries. As a large group, receive any comments about the exercise.

Note

Some pairs may need help to encourage A to elaborate. It is a good idea to walk around the class, prompting where necessary.

Exercise 6.2 Functions of questions

Time

Homework (can be done with Exercise 6.3) plus 'marking' and short follow-up session.

Preparation

1. Copies of Table 6.1 for every student.
2. Instructions and answer sheets for every student.

Organization

1. Issue students with copies of Table 6.1 and ask them to collect examples of five questions from work/school settings and five questions from home/social settings.
2. Collect the lists of questions and check them for appropriate matching with functions. Set date for follow-up session. (An alternative to the tutor 'marking' the lists is to ask students to 'mark' each other's.)
3. In follow-up session return students' work to them and as a large group consider the discussion issues.

Note

If Exercise 6.3 is done at the same time, discuss both exercises together.

Exercise 6.3 Open and closed questions

Time

45 minutes plus optional homework (can be done with Exercise 6.2).

Preparation

1. If Exercise 6.2 was completed, students are to bring their list of questions collected. If not, provide students with a list of 10 questions used by nurses. The questions should, ideally, differ in style.
2. Instructions and answer sheets for every student.
3. If homework is to be done, enough answer sheets for every student.

Organization

1. Ask students to write out their list of questions on the answer sheet, and to 'transcribe' them into open and closed formats.
2. Divide the class into pairs to 'check' each others' answers.
3. Combine to the large group and consider the discussion issues.
4. Homework (optional): Issue answer sheets. Either arrange to collect the completed sheets for checking, or organize the students to check each other's charts.

Note

There should be no problems conducting this exercise.

Exercise 6.4 Giving information

Time

1–1½ hours

Preparation

1. Copies of Figures 6.1 and 6.2 for every student.
2. Large sheets of paper, felt tip markers and blue tac or similar for each group of four.
3. Instructions and answer sheets for every student.

Organization

1. In groups of four distribute copies of Figures 6.1 and 6.2, answer sheets, and large sheets of paper.
2. Ask each group to devise an explanation for a different topic. As far as possible, do not use a topic of which the group members have no experience.
3. Ask each group to list the major points of explanation on the large sheets of paper to show to the whole class.
4. After 20–30 minutes call a stop and reconvene the large group. Ask each group in turn to announce their topic and display their list of points. They should then give their piece of information to the class.
5. After each presentation discuss the information with reference to Figures 6.1 and 6.2 and to the discussion issues.

Note

There should be no problems conducting this exercise.

Exercise 6.5 Jargon and technical language

Time

Homework plus half hour follow-up

Preparation

Instructions and answer sheets for every student.

Organization

1. Issue students with instructions and answer sheets and request that they complete them (individually or in collaboration). Give a date for follow-up session.
2. In follow-up session, in groups of six, hear each other's re-writes and discuss them in relation to the discussion issues.
3. Conclude session by asking the large group if there were any issues arising from their discussions they wished to pursue.

Note

Some students may not have completed their homework. Try to ensure that they do not feel they can just rely on others in the group. It may be an idea to group those who have not done the homework together and ask them to re-write the explanations during the session. A reminder to the group of the importance of homework may be necessary.

Exercise 6.6 Deficiencies in giving information

Time

45 minutes

Preparation

Instructions and answer sheets for every student.

Organization

1. Issue all students with instructions and answer sheets. Ask them to complete the answer sheets individually or in collaboration. Allow 15 minutes.
2. Reconvene the large group and summarize the deficiencies detected by the class in the following categories:

   (a) Process of giving information:

   (i) Needs
   (ii) Checking
   (iii) Planning
   (iv) Presenting
   (v) Concluding

 (b) Medium used.
 (c) Jargon and technical language.
 (d) Style of question.

3. Consider the discussion issues.

Note

There should be no problems conducting this exercise.

Exercise 6.7 Assertion, aggression, passivity and manipulation

Time

Either homework plus 20-minute follow-up session or 1 hour.

Preparation

1. Copies of Table 6.3 and instructions and answer sheets for each person.
2. Case study of mishandled situation (in reserve — see Note below).

Organization

1. If homework, ask each student to complete the answer sheet individually. If used as class exercise, in groups of four, ask each member to choose a situation during the last week that she/he would have liked to have handled more assertively, and to complete the answer sheet. Set date for follow-up session. During this session clarify the nature of assertion.
2. Groups choose the example they found the most interesting to relate to the class.
3. Reconvene the large group and hear the examples. Invite the class to question what did/could have happened. Consider the discussion issues.

Note

Some students may not be able to think of examples. In case the whole class is unable/unwilling to give instances, it is a good idea to have a 'case study' available for general discussion.

Exercise 6.8 Levels of assertion

Time

Homework plus short follow-up session.

Preparation

Instructions and answer sheets for every student.

Organization

1. Ask students to complete the inventory. They may do it individually or with discussion. Set date for follow-up session.
2. *Follow-up:* Briefly consider any problems that arose in the homework, or in the consideration of the discussion issues.

Note

If students are unsure of the meaning of any of the items in the questionnaire, they should exclude them.

Exercise 6.9 Being specific

Time

15 minutes

Preparation

Instructions and answer sheets for every student.

Organization

1. Issue instructions and answer sheets and ask students to complete them individually.
2. As a large group, discuss instances where being specific is difficult. Summarize these situations on the board in the light of the discussion issues.

Note

There should be no problem conducting this exercise.

Exercise 6.10 Broken record: fielding responses

Time

$2\frac{1}{2}$ hours or two sessions of $1\frac{1}{2}$ hours

Preparation

Sets of instructions for each student.

Organization

1. Divide the class into groups of three and allocate roles A, B and C. Issue each person with instructions.
2. After 45 minutes, at the end of the first part of the exercise, reconvene the large group and consider briefly students' experiences during this part of the exercise. Discuss some of the consequences of sticking to the point.
3. Repeat the exercise with reference to *fielding responses*.
4. After a further 45 minutes, reconvene the large group and consider briefly students' experiences during this part of the exercise. Discuss some of the consequences of fielding responses.

Note

A may find it hard to brief B about her/his role. It does not matter if the role play does not mirror what happened in the original situation. Encourage A to give as much background information as possible. C may need some help in advising A and B. Tutor might need to circulate among the groups in order to assist. Students often find it difficult to stick to the task. Tutors should check that all groups are following the instructions.

Exercise 6.11 Dealing with criticism

Time

45 minutes

Preparation

Instructions and answer sheets for every student.

Organization

1. In pairs, ask students to complete the answer sheets.
2. Combine in groups of six and discuss one example from each person from Section B. Group members should try to improve the assertive reply if possible.
3. In the groups of six, consider the discussion issues.
4. Conclude session by drawing out the implications of this exercise for giving constructive (and assertive) criticism.

Note

There should be no problems conducting this exercise.

Exercise 6.12 Receiving and giving compliments

Time

45 minutes

Preparation

1. Instructions and answer sheets for every student.
2. Large sheets of paper, felt markers, blue tac or similar.

Organization

1. In pairs, ask students to complete the answer sheets.
2. Combine to groups of four and allow 10 minutes to discuss the exercise in relation to the discussion issues. Ask groups to list four factors that affect the ease of giving and receiving compliments, in order to display around the room.
3. Display the poster summaries around the room and invite students to examine them.
4. Conclude session by drawing attention to similarities/dissimilarities in the factors produced.

Note

There should be no problems with this exercise, although a lot of giggling might occur during Section B. Many students find this task difficult and sometimes stressful: it is a lot easier in class situations to criticize others than to compliment them. Use this as a point for discussion.

Chapter 7

Exercise 7.1 Identification of goals and alternative strategies

Time

$1\frac{1}{2}$ hours

Preparation

1. At least three samples of video-taped interactions of about six minutes each. These should, if possible, be of nursing situations (see Appendix III for examples of video-taped material).
2. Video replay equipment.
3. Instructions and answer sheets for every student to complete for each scene.

Organization

1. Issue students with instructions and answer sheets.
2. Split class into groups of four.
3. Show one scene and allow students 10 minutes to discuss the scene and to complete the answer sheet.
4. Repeat for each scene.
5. Reconvene the large group to consider the discussion issues.
6. Conclude with brief discussion of constraints that are imposed on 'ideal' ways of dealing with interpersonal problems.

Note

There should be no problems conducting this exercise. Some groups may wish for longer discussions.

Exercise 7.2 Social problem solving

Time

1–1½ hours

Preparation

1. Copies of Figure 7.1 for every student.
2. Instructions and answer sheets for every student.

Organization

1. Split class into groups of four or five. Issue copies of Figure 7.1 and answer sheets.
2. Ask each group to work through the problems as instructed and to generate a further 'problem' that they have met at work, in order to present a social problem solving analysis of it to the whole class. Ask them to bear in mind the discussion issues as they do this.
3. Hear each group's case study. Make sure that all stages of the social problem solving process have been covered. If some are difficult to incorporate, use this as the basis of discussion.
4. Conclude session by pointing to the complexities of interpersonal situations that would emerge if everyone were to use a social problem solving approach. Consider whether the approach is useful for understanding/dealing with interpersonal conflicts.

Note

There should be no difficulties with this exercise, but the tutor must be familiar with the social problem solving approach.

Exercise 7.3 The development of attitudes

Time

Homework plus 20 minutes follow-up.

Preparation

Instructions and answer sheets for every student.

Organization

1. Issue students with instructions and answer sheets and ask them to complete them as homework either by themselves or in discussion. Ask students to bring their completed sheets to the follow-up session (set date).
2. *Follow-up:* Consider any difficulties students had in doing the task, and briefly consider the discussion issues.
3. Conclude with reference to the role of different socializing agents in the development of attitudes.

Note

Some students may not have done their homework. Emphasize the collective responsibility for doing homework. If appropriate, split the class into those that have and have not done the homework for the discussions. Do not let those who have not done it 'ride' on those that have.

Exercise 7.4 The meaning of prejudice

Time

Homework plus 1 hour follow-up.

Preparation

1. Instructions and diagrams for every student.
2. For follow-up session, large sheets of paper, felt markers and blue tac or similar.

Organization

1. Issue all students with instructions and answer sheets. Set date for follow-up session.
2. *Follow-up:* Combine in groups of six. Issue each group with discussion issues, large sheets of paper and felt markers. Ask each group to prepare a summary diagram from the individual homework pieces, entitled 'Prejudice in Nursing'. Allow 30 minutes.
3. Display the summary diagrams around the room and invite the class to examine them.

4. Summarize session by drawing out the persistent themes relating to the development, nature and change of prejudice in nursing arising from the posters.

Note

Some students may not like to think of themselves as being prejudiced at all and may be distressed to find themselves the 'objects' of other people's prejudices. It may help to join the group discussions for short periods, and help students confront their prejudices. Tutors should be prepared to reveal some of their own prejudices and to be familiar with the general theoretical field (see Further Reading Chapter 7).

Exercise 7.5 Cognitive dissonance and attitude change

Time

1 hour

Preparation

Instructions and answer sheets for every student.

Organization

1. Distribute instruction and answer sheets and ask students to complete them in pairs.
2. Reconvene the large group and ask for one example from each pair. Discuss these as they are presented with reference to the discussion issues.
3. Conclude with a revision of the role of dissonance in attitude change.

Note

It is necessary for students to understand the concept of cognitive dissonance in order to carry out this exercise. Some reminder may be necessary. Students may balk at the label 'cognitive dissonance'. The label is not important but the concept is.

Exercise 7.6 Persuasive appeals

Time

2 hours or more, depending on the number of groups.

Preparation

1. Copies of Table 7.1 for all students.
2. Instructions to read or distribute to all students.
3. Plenty of paper, pens, sellotape, and other 'props' as necessary.

Organization

1. Split the class into groups of 4–8 people. Issue all students with copies of Table 7.1, and instructions.
2. Ask each group to prepare their persuasive appeal to deliver to the rest of the class, paying due consideration to the factors summarized in Table 7.1. The appeal may take any form, and be enacted with reference to any channel. It should take about 5–10 minutes to deliver.
3. Groups may choose their own topics. This can be anything they are likely to be involved with as nurses. If some groups cannot think of titles, use one from the examples given in the exercise.
4. After 30 minutes of planning, hear/see each group's presentation. Ask each group to run quickly over the decisions they made in planning their appeal.
5. Conclude the session by reiterating both the social problem solving process and the decisions to be made in devising persuasive appeals.

Note

This exercise is intended to be (and usually is) light-hearted. Encourage students to be creative in their attempts at persuasion. Take care, though, to extract the importance of the decisions that were made from the finished products.

Chapter 8

Exercise 8.1 Counselling and other helping relationships

Time

1½ hours

Preparation

1. Instructions and answer sheets for every student.
2. A definition of counselling for distribution or presentation on overhead projector.

Organization

1. Ask students, in pairs, to complete the first section of the answer sheet. Allow 10 minutes.
2. Combine into groups of four in order to construct a definition of counselling. Allow 10 minutes.
3. Combine in groups of 8 in order to write down all the problems, worries or issues that patients, relatives and colleagues have brought to the members recently. Consider the discussion issues and tick those problems for which counselling would be an appropriate form of helping. Ask each group to select one example to relate to the class. Allow 30–40 minutes.
4. Reconvene the large group and hear each example. Consider whether counselling would, indeed, have been appropriate.
5. Conclude by offering a definition of counselling.

Note

Ideally, students should have had some input on the nature of counselling prior to doing this exercise. Some groups may get stuck thinking of examples and may need prompting.

Exercise 8.2 Exploration: clarifying and understanding

Time

Homework plus 1 hour follow-up.

Preparation

1. Instructions for all students.
2. Large sheets of paper, felt markers and blue tac or similar for each group of 4–6.

Organization

1. Issue students with the instructions to do as a homework exercise. Ask them to bring their examples to the follow-up session (set date).
2. *Follow-up:* Divide the class in groups of 4–6. Issue each group with a large sheet of paper and felt markers. Ask students to discuss their examples and to choose the one they think is the best illustration for presentation to the class. Ask each group to write their example on the large sheet of paper.
3. Display the examples around the room and invite students to circulate and to read them.
4. Reconvene the large group and consider the discussion issues.

Note

Some students may not have done their homework. Do not mix them with those who have, but ask them to generate examples in the class. Stress the importance and collective responsibility of doing homework.

Exercise 8.3 Descriptions of feelings

Time

1 hour (or more)

Preparation

Instructions and answer sheets for all students.

Organization

1. Divide the class into groups of four and ask them to complete the exercise. Ask each group to choose one colloquialism over which there was most disagreement/ignorance about to relate to the class.
2. Reconvene the large group and hear the examples chosen by the groups.
3. Summarize the discussion by highlighting the problems of using inappropriate metaphor/colloquialism for capturing the essence of other people's expression of feelings.

Note

This exercise could be done as homework, although a lot is gained through group discussion. A variation might be to display the lists of colloquialisms on large sheets of paper around the classroom. At times there may be disagreement as to the meaning of colloquial statements, and the tutor may be asked to adjudicate. She/he may not be familiar with the expression, in which case she/he should acknowledge this, but draw out the implications of a lack of common understanding of such phrases for nursing practice.

Exercise 8.4 Paraphrasing and reflecting

Time

1 hour plus homework plus 1½ hour follow-up.

Preparation

Instructions and answer sheets for every student and for homework.

Organization

1. *Session 1:* Inform class of the three stages to the exercise. Give dates for all sessions.
2. Divide the class into pairs and ask each pair to work through the paraphrasing section of the exercise.
3. Reconvene the large group and have a short discussion on how easy/hard the paraphrasing was.
4. Ask students to complete the further paraphrasing section as homework, giving date for follow-up session.
5. *Follow-up:* Check with the class for difficulties in doing the homework and discuss them.
6. Divide the class into small groups (5/6) and ask them to complete the reflecting part of the exercise.
7. Ask all groups to discuss the exercise with reference to the discussion issues.
8. Reconvene the large group and have brief discussion about the difficulties of paraphrasing/reflecting. Summarize these difficulties on the board, in terms of (a) personal, (b) organizational difficulties. End the session by emphasizing the central role of paraphrasing and reflecting for person-centred counselling.

Note

Each part of this exercise depends on the others, so everything possible should be done to ensure that students participate in all parts. The second session can be conducted in pairs: the group exercise sometimes encourages students to be flippant. Careful tutor monitoring of groups may be necessary. It is possible that students may get emotionally involved in what they are talking about. Care should be taken to ensure that students are all 'de-roled' before leaving the class.

Exercise 8.5 Concreteness: general to specific

Time

Homework plus 1-hour follow-up.

Preparation

Instructions and answer sheets for every student.

Organization

1. Distribute instructions and answer sheets and ask students to complete them prior to the follow-up session. Set date for follow-up session.
2. *Follow-up:* In pairs, allocate roles A and B and issue the following instructions:

   A — Please make a general statement about an experience you have had recently. Try to include how it *felt* as well as what happened.

   B — Please try to get A to be more specific through the use of questions. For example: A — 'Lots of meetings have been cancelled and I've got quite annoyed.' B — 'Can you tell me exactly what it feels like?' *or* 'Will you describe the last time it happened?' etc.

   Swop roles and repeat.
3. Ask pairs to discuss their experiences in the light of discussion issues.
4. Hear some pairs' examples of situations requiring them to encourage concreteness in their nursing practice. Briefly discuss the disadvantages of non-specificity or generalizing.

Note

There should be no problems conducting this exercise. Some students may not have done their homework. Those students should be asked to do the homework in class time.

Exercise 8.6 Summarizing to move conversations on

Time

1 hour

Preparation

1. Table 8.2 to distribute to all students.
2. Instructions and answer sheets for all students.

Organization

1. In groups of four, construct replies to each of the examples, as instructed.
2. Reconvene the large group and hear one example of a summary from each small group.
3. Briefly consider the discussion issues as a large group, and summarize the major themes on the board.

Note

Some groups may need help in clarifying the differences between the different forms of summary.

Exercise 8.7 Identification of personal strengths

Time

1 hour

Preparation

Instructions for every student.

Organization

1. In pairs ask students to work through the instructions.
2. Reconvene the large group and hold a brief discussion about barriers in nursing that prevent people using their personal strengths to best effect. Note that the focusing on positive characteristics of our own or of others is not encouraged in western society, and discuss why this might be.

Note

Students may find this exercise difficult and may need prompting.

Exercise 8.8 Setting realistic goals

Time

1 hour

Preparation

1. Instructions and goal-setting charts for every student.
2. Large sheets of paper, felt markers and blue tac or similar.

Organization

1. Issue all students with goal-setting charts. Ask them to work through them individually.
2. In pairs, choose one aim and explore with each other how this aim could be turned into a manageable, realistic goal that could be achieved in the near future.
3. Ask each pair to choose one goal-setting chart to display on posters for the class.
4. Display the posters and invite all students to look at them.
5. Reconvene the large group and consider the discussion issues. Summarize the main points on the board.

Note

There should be no problems conducting this exercise.

Exercise 8.9 Brainstorming

Time

1½ hours

Preparation

Instructions for every group of 4–6.

Organization

1. Split class into groups of six. Issue each group with the instructions.
2. Ask each group to choose one problem to present the solutions they considered to the whole class.
3. After allowing plenty of time for lots of solutions to be generated for each problem, reconvene the large group. Ask each small group to give their most and least preferred solutions to their chosen problem.
4. Consider the discussion issues.

Note

This exercise can be noisy as groups think of creative and often fantastic solutions to the problems. This should be encouraged.

Exercise 8.10 Force-field analysis

Time

1½ hours

Preparation

1. Copies of Figure 8.2 for all students.
2. Instructions and force-field analysis charts for all students.

Organization

1. Issue all students with instructions and copies of Figure 8.2.
2. Divide the class into pairs and ask them to work through the force-field analyses as instructed.
3. Reconvene the large group to consider the dicussion issues.

Note

Some students may find the task difficult. They may not be able to think of a problem that would be suitable for the force-field analysis. Point out that all problems can be subjected to force-field analyses. However, it is a good idea to have some 'problems' to hand to give to students if they really cannot think of one of their own. Mix with the class to help pairs in difficulty.

Chapter 9

Exercise 9.1 Development of relationships

Time

Homework plus 45-minute follow-up.

Preparation

1. Instructions and answer sheets for every student.
2. Discussion issues to distribute/present on overhead projectors.

Organization

1. Issue all students with questionnaires.
2. Ask students to complete the questionnaire individually at home and to bring to follow-up session (give date).
3. *Follow-up:* Combine in groups of six and ask each group to prepare a summary of which aspect of relationships with patients are similar to those of (a) close friends and (b) professional colleagues. Ask them to list similarities:

   Relationships with patients have the following similarities with:
   Close friends   *Professional colleagues*

4. After 15 minutes reconvene large group, hear each group's summaries and combine them in two lists on the board/overhead projector.
5. Consider briefly the discussion points and conclude by drawing attention to the particular (often stressful) qualities of relationships with patients.

Note

There should be no difficulties conducting this exercise. Some students may not have done their homework. Group these students together and ask them to fill in the questionnaire during class time. Try not to let them 'ride' on the work of others. Emphasize the collective responsibility of doing homework.

Exercise 9.2 Professional support systems

Time

1½–2 hours

Preparation

1. Instructions and answer sheets for every student.
2. Paper and pencils.
3. Discussion issues to distribute/present on overhead projector.

Organization

1. In groups of six, issue each group with sets of instructions. Ask the groups to elect 'scribes' and 'presenters'. Issue instructions.
2. Allow 45 minutes for groups to prepare their cases.
3. Reconvene large group and invite presenters to read out their 'cases'.
4. Discuss each 'case' briefly in the light of discussion points.
5. Conclude session by exploring ways that students can establish their own support groups.

Note

Some students may think their own support systems are adequate. Ask them to write a summary of how their support systems operate, illustrating its advantages and disadvantages with reference to the guidelines.

Exercise 9.3 The influence of liking and disliking on interpersonal skills

Time

1½ hours

Preparation

1. Instructions and answer sheets for every student.
2. Large sheets of paper and felt markers.

Organization

1. Working individually complete answer sheets (allow 30 minutes.)
2. In pairs, consider similarities in how patients who are liked and disliked are dealt with. Ask pairs to list the similarities on a large sheet of paper (allow 20 minutes).
3. Display lists around the room and invite students to circulate and read them (10 minutes).
4. Reconvene large group. Draw out common interpersonal themes from the posters and briefly consider discussion issues.

Note

There should be no problems in conducting the exercise although some students may claim not to dislike patients at all. Suggest they think about *relative* liking and disliking.

Exercise 9.4 Regulations

Time

1 hour

Preparation

Instructions and answer sheets for every student.

Organization

1. Ask students to complete the answer sheets working individually.
2. Combine in pairs. Ask these pairs to generate more examples if possible and to consider the discussion issues. Ask each pair to choose one example to relate to the class.
3. Reconvene the large group and hear each example. Summarize the constraints imposed on the use of interpersonal skill that emerge.
4. Conclude session by considering any positive ways that regulations can influence the interpersonal skills of nurses.

Note

There should be no problems conducting this exercise.

Exercise 9.5 Organizational constraints on the use of interpersonal skills

Time

1 hour

Preparation

Instructions and answer sheets for every student.

Organization

1. Ask students to consider the answer sheets, working individually.
2. Combine in pairs. Ask these pairs to generate more examples if possible and to consider the discussion issues. Ask each pair to choose one example to relate to the class.
3. Reconvene the large group and hear each example. Summarize the constraints imposed on the use of interpersonal skill that emerge.
4. Conclude session by considering any positive ways that organizational factors can influence the interpersonal skills of nurses.

Note

There should be no problems conducting this exercise.

Exercise 9.6 Environmental constraints on the use of interpersonal skills: physical features

Time

Homework plus 1-hour follow-up.

Preparation

Instructions and answer sheets for every student.

Organization

1. *Homework:* Ask students to prepare maps of a nursing setting and to bring them to the follow-up session (set date).
2. *Follow up:* In pairs, consider the maps that have been drawn and identify ways in which interpersonal skills are constrained (directly and indirectly) by physical features of the setting. Ask each pair to note the feature they think has the greatest constraining effect on the use of interpersonal skills to report to the class and to consider the discussion issues.
3. Reconvene the large group and ask each pair for their most salient feature. Summarize on the board or overhead projector.
4. Conclude session by discussing ways in which the physical environment might be overcome.

Note

Some students may not have done their homework, in which case they should be encouraged to complete the task in class time. The whole exercise could be done in class time. A further homework/class exercise could be to design an 'ideal' physcial nursing setting.

Exercise 9.7 Environmental constraints on the use of interpersonal skills: thwartings

Time

Homework plus 1-hour follow-up.

Preparation

Answer sheets for every student.

Organization

1. *Homework:* Ask students to prepare maps of a nursing setting and to bring them to the follow-up session (set date). Maps for Exercise 9.6 may be used again.
2. *Follow-up:* In pairs, consider the maps that have been drawn and identify ways in which interpersonal skills are constrained (directly and indirectly) by those features over which people have no control, or 'thwartings'. Ask

each pair to note the feature they think has the greatest constraining effect to report to the class, and to consider the discussion issues.
3. Reconvene the large group and ask each pair for their most salient feature. Summarize on the board or overhead projector.
4. Conclude session by discussing ways in which such 'thwartings' might be overcome.

Note

Some students may not have done their homework, in which case they should be encouraged to complete the task in class time. The whole exercise could be done in class time. A further homework/class exercise could be to design an 'ideal' environment that minimized the number of 'thwartings'.

Exercise 9.8 Cultural constraints and the use of interpersonal skills

Time

Homework plus $1\frac{1}{2}$ hours.

Preparation

1. Instructions and answer sheets for every student.
2. Large sheets of paper, felt markers, blue tac or similar.

Organization

1. Divide class into four. Allocate each section a media source to analyze for its representation of health, illness and nursing. Examples are:
   (a) Different Sunday newspapers on the same day.
   (b) Specified television documentary/soap opera.
   (c) Specified radio feature/documentary/play.
   (d) Specified feature film.
   (e) Selection of women's magazines (past/present; for different readerships, etc.)
2. Issue question sheets to be completed as homework to bring to the follow-up session (set date).
3. *Follow-up:* In groups of 3–6, all of whom had the same source to investigate, compare notes and consider the discussion issues. Ask group to prepare a summary to relate to the whole class (40 minutes).

4. Reconvene large group and hear each group's summary and put major points on the board separately for each media source.
5. Summarize the 'messages' of different media sources.
6. Discuss the implications of the findings for individuals in different nursing contexts. Consider further discussion issues:

Further discussion issues

1. Do cultural factors influence the interpersonal skills of nurses in some nursing contexts more than others? How?
2. What is the greatest contemporary challenge to nurses in the current social/cultural context?
3. Conclude session by discussing briefly the role of nurses in bringing about social/political change and link this to the ways they can/cannot use interpersonal skills.

Note

This exercise can bring about heated exchanges. Students can be made aware of their own positions and the importance of this for self-awareness. Tutors, too, have views and it is important to emphasize that there are no right/wrong answers to any of the questions.

The media 'sampling' can vary. It is particularly interesting to look at historical material. Public libraries and old newspapers etc. are a good source.

Chapter 10

Exercises 10.1–10.4

Time

Variable. Time should be set at the start of every role play.

Preparation

1. Statements of the objectives of the particular role play (for example, 'To gain insight into some of the social forces brought to bear on people who are dependent on others; to experience a conflict between expectations and actual behaviour; to explore different ways of resolving role strain, etc.').

2. Copies of role 'scripts' for all participants.
3. Props (such as blindfolds) as necessary.
4. Discussion issues to distribute at the end of each role play.

Organization

1. Introduce the session by stating the objectives of the particular role play (it can sometimes be useful to display the objectives on a notice board, so the session can be evaluated with respect to them at the end).
2. Split the class into pairs/small groups and allocate the roles and scripts. Clarify any guidelines to be followed (such as 'Do not discuss your scripts with each other' etc.).
3. Clarify any concerns the participants have, and set a time limit. Make it quite clear whether the role plays are to be conducted 'publicly' with the rest of the class watching, privately in the classroom, or 'in vivo'. If the role play is to be recorded on audio or video tape, ensure that participants know this and that they have agreed to it.
4. Ensure that all participants are thoroughly de-roled after the role play. It can sometimes be necessary for participants to 'rehearse' some aspects of their real life roles, in order to bring them back to reality.
5. Leave plenty of time for all those involved to discuss the experiences of the role play, and to consider whether the objectives of the session were met through the role play. Invite suggestions as to how they might be better met.

Note

Some students may be reluctant to take part in role play. Generally, students will derive little benefit if they are coerced to participate.

Some role plays may be difficult for some students to take seriously. It is a good idea to discuss with them how a role play could be structured more appropriately. Some students, though, may just get the 'uncontrollable giggles'. Little can be done about this, although there is never any benefit in a tutor getting annoyed with them. It is best to be tolerant, and to try to see the funny side!

Some role plays may lead students to become engrossed in the role. This is especially true of those that contain a lot of emotional content. Tutors must be able to handle these incidents sensitively, and to know when to call a halt to an activity. All students should be thoroughly de-roled before leaving the classroom: this may mean that some students have to be asked to stay behind for additional de-roling. Occasionally students may need some specialist knowledge to play a role meaningfully. Tutors should ensure that this is available or that the role play is adapted for the particular students involved.

APPENDIX II

ADDITIONAL INFORMATION FOR THE EXERCISES

Exercise 3.15 Reconstruction of memory

Messages

1. Every morning you'll receive a bottle. Do a sample and leave it on the table round the corner by the time the drinks come round. Keep a note of the capacity — the bottles are calibrated along the sides.
2. Put three drops in both ears, twice a day, for about four days. Use cotton wool if it leaks out. Store it at room temperature. Lay her on her front, and we'll see her again in a week or so.
3. We'll do two weeks as you are, then two weeks with the increased Beclaforte four times a day. And in addition we'll then do two weeks on the Atrovent as well as the Ventolin, Beclaforte and 450 Phyllocontin twice a day. This will be a scientific way to go about it, and we'll see how you go.
4. She has long sight in both eyes and a slight astigmatism in the right. Her left is dragging a bit — what we call a lazy eye. So we must make it do some work. Here are some occlusion patches. Try to make her wear it on the right for about half an hour a day. Collect some more as you need

them. I'll give you a prescription for the glasses to be made up at the opticians. Don't rush her — she won't like it. Be thinking of building up to 3–4 hours in 6 months. For close work. Then you'll be doing well.

Exercise 4.2 Group identification

Over the period 1980–85, students from these groups have scored the following averages on the same task:

Psychiatric nurses	32
Social workers	34
Youth and community workers	36
Medical students	36
Psychology students	37
Sociology students	37
Accountancy students	38
Law students	38
English students	40
Physiotherapists	40

Discussion issues

1. Why was there an increase in the numbers detected? Was the observation that the other group did better an influence on performance?
2. What went through your mind as you approached the task the second time?
3. Would the effect have been lesser/greater if your score had been compared with any other group? Why?
4. Are there any situations in nursing where comparison with another group leads to group cohesion/competitiveness/individual identity with the group?
5. Can this process be used to help patients get better, wards to run more efficiently, etc.? How?

Exercise 5.2 Expression and recognition of emotion

Contradictory messages

(a) Well, Mrs Robinson, I'm so pleased you're feeling better. (*Sad.*)
(b) Oh come now, Nurse Briggs, I've told you dozens of times how to do it! (*Surprise.*)
(c) I hear you had a jolly good talk with Dr Evans? (*Fear.*)
(d) I don't like to leave you alone in this state. (*Disgust.*)
(e) I think that's a revolting thing to have done! (*Happy.*)
(f) It's such a shame you've got to move to the other ward. (*Anger.*)

Exercise 6.1 Speech elicitation

Instructions for person B

When your partners return, please ask them to tell you about their experiences. Tell them that they have 20 minutes in which to do this. They will, of course, not be able to talk for this long, and will probably dry up fairly quickly. Your task is to try to get them to talk for as long as possible about their time out of the room. Encourage them as much as you can. Try to get them to elaborate what they tell you — to describe exactly what they did, saw, heard, smelt, felt, as well as what they thought about the experience. Ask them about their thoughts and feelings; about any smells and sensations they experienced; about textures of walls, floors, colours, other people, associations with past events, and so on.

Exercise 10.3 Role conflict through differing expectations and excessive demands: Role scripts

The 'rights' of elderly people (1)

Person B — Community nurse

B — You are a community nurse who has been involved with Mrs Campbell, a 76-year-old widow who lives alone, for quite some time. She has recently been told by the orthoptist that surgical treatment of her cataracts would help her vision Mrs. Campbell is reluctant to go into hospital and is convinced that her failing sight is due to 'old age', and that she should accept it. Her daughter has told you that the family are encouraging Mrs Campbell to have the surgery and that she will take little persuasion. You have been asked by the G.P. to see Mrs Campbell with a view to agreeing a date to discuss admission.

Task

You aim to get Mrs Campbell to agree to discuss being admitted for surgery.

The 'rights' of elderly people (2)

Person B — Elderly patient

B — you are a 67-year-old man who has just had a hip replacement. You are due to go home today. You have had enough of medical personnel and want to be left alone when you go home. You do not want the district nurse to call on you and you threaten not to open the door if she/he does. You have a daughter who lives nearby who will do your shopping for you. You are convinced that the new hip will be no better then the previous one, so there is no point trying to 'get it going'.

Task

You want to be assured that no more nursing staff will bother you when you get home. You try to get this assurance from the staff nurse.

Conflicting concerns

Person B — Ward sister

B — your ward operates a policy of trying to ensure that all your patients fully understand the nature of their illnesses and of any medical techniques that are to be applied to them. A new patient, a 42-year-old woman, has been admitted for investigations into a recurrent stomach problem. The likelihood is that she has a growth. At any rate, the tests she will have to undergo will be unpleasant and you wish (a) to make her feel comfortable about being in hospital and (b) fully to prepare her for the ensuing tests.

Task

You try to make her feel comfortable, but more importantly to prepare her for the tests.

Professional rivalry

Person B — S.E.N.

B — you are a 38-year-old S.E.N. who has been working on the children's ward for 14 years. You have seen many staff come and go and know the routine very well. Recently a new staff nurse has been appointed who has far less experience of nursing than you. He appears, in your view to be more interested in moving up the career ladder than in nursing. You feel hostile and 'bristly' every time he comes to talk to you. You feel he will 'walk all over you' to further his own careerist ends at every opportunity. You always make sure that he appreciates just how much more experienced than him you are.

Task

You have always been one of the nurses doing the drugs when you are on duty. The new staff nurse refuses to have you (an S.E.N.) involved. You try to make him see 'sense'.

Professional boundaries

Person B — Male patient

B — you are Mr Foster, aged 52. You have been in hospital for three weeks and have struck up a good friendship with one of the student nurses. She has said on many occasions that she would do anything for you — you only have to ask. During your stay in hospital you have not had any visitors, even though your daughter and her family live nearby. You feel it must be because for some reason your daughter does not know you are in hospital, even though the ward clerk assures you that she has been notified. You decide to ask the nurse to call on your daughter to ask her to visit you. You are sure she (the nurse) will not mind.

Task

You try to arrange for the nurse to see your daughter.

Competing roles

Person B — Student nurse

B — you are a student nurse who is in the middle of the psychiatry block. You have been asked to take a history from a patient who has been admitted earlier in the day. The patient is confused and has had some psychotic incidents. To your dismay you find that the patient is one of your close circle of friends. Unbeknown to any of you she has been in and out of hospital for the last three years.

Task

You have to try to overcome the embarrassment you both feel, and set the 'ground rules' for your relationship in the hospital.

Personal limitations

Person B — Patient

B — you are a young mother of three who was admitted to the Accident and Emergency Department last night following an overdose. You had fully intended to kill yourself as you cannot cope with your life any more, and feel that everyone would be better off if you were dead. This morning you wake up on the female medical ward. The last thing you want is to be treated gingerly and any attempts to do this are met with impatience. You want to make it quite clear to everyone you come in contact with that you will try to kill yourself again at the earliest opportunity. As soon as you feel strong enough you will discharge yourself.

Task

You have to ensure that any of the nurses who come near you understand your position.

Resource limitations

Person B — District nurse

B — you are a district nurse who is calling on a 48-year-old woman with multiple sclerosis. She is severely handicapped and wheelchair bound. You have been nursing her for some time, and have a good relationship. This morning she is due for her weekly bath. She lives in a specially adapted flat. It is midsummer and very hot: there is little ventilation in the flat. Mrs Barnett is usually good humoured, but today she is crotchety, expressing the desire for daily baths. You sympathize with her, but know that the district nurse service cannot stretch to this.

Task

Negotiate over the bath issue.

APPENDIX III

RESOURCES: A BRIEF INTRODUCTION

Resources

Pictures, films, audio/video tapes, television programmes, novels, short stories and activities can all be used to 'trigger' discussion, insight and experience, and are, therefore, valuable aids to interpersonal skills teaching.

We list below some sources of materials that we have worked with and found useful. We do not think it is useful to use any of these materials in place of tutors, even in cases where the product is marketed as a 'complete learning system'. We have found, instead, that they are all of more value as just one part of a teaching programme. In our experience, careful monitoring through discussion, with a tutor present, highlights learning issues, and provides the vital links between the 'trigger' material and the context in which students live and work.

This is only a selection of resources. Most libraries can obtain catalogues of film and video material, and give advice on how to build up a useful audio/visual collection. Nevertheless, we hope you find something of interest here.

General

Concord Films Council
201 Felixstow Road
Ipswich

Catalogue of films and videos for hire.

Audio tapes

Talking to Patients 27 minutes (1969)
Various issues concerned with communication, including verbal strategies, expressions, actions, finding time.

The Importance of Good Communication 35 minutes (1978)
Focuses on the elderly and others with whom communication is difficult.

Available from:
Graves Medical AV Library
Holly House
220 New London Road
Chelmsford, Essex
CM2 9BJ
0245 83351

Principles of Counselling (F. Inskipp and H. Johns)
I — four cassettes with notes and exercises (1983).
II — four cassettes with notes and exercises (1985).
Based on BBC series of same title. Manual for trainers written by F. Inskipp also available.

Available from:
Alexia Publications
2 Market Terrace
St Leonards-on-Sea
East Sussex
TN38 0DB
0424 427948

Video tapes

Breaking Bad News 30 minutes
Two simulated encounters between doctors and relatives. Highlights important aspects of talking to relatives, including the need to assess the amount of information that is known and that can be handled. Raises questions relating to the setting in which the news is given. Discussion breaks.

Handling Difficult Questions 30 minutes
Examines a micro-teaching system for helping a specialist nurse respond to patients who have not been told the truth about their condition. Discussion breaks.

Depression: Understanding and Helping 57 minutes
Role-played crisis situation. Suggestions for how to work with a depressed client highlighting the importance of listening and support for helpers. Discussion breaks.

Available from:
Tavistock Publications Ltd   — *there are many other titles on*
11 New Fetter Lane   *their distribution list*
London
EC4P 4EE

Communication in Patient Care
Samples of live nurse–patient interactions in different settings (background noise included!) Tutor/student notes supplied.
1. *Talking with the Cancer Patient*
2. *Talking with the Geriatric Patient*
3. *Talking with the Stoma Care Patient*
4. *Talking with Children in Hospital*

Available from:
Abbott Laboratories Ltd   *or* Macmillan Publishers Ltd
Queensborough   Houndmills
Sheerness   Basingstoke
Kent   Hants
ME11 5EL   RG21 2JQ
0799 663371   0256 29243

Listening and Responding: Counselling Skills in Nursing Care (M. Conner, G. Dexter and M. Wash)
Manual for tutors with three video modules. Introductory level: suitable for initial nurse training.

Available from:
Eduational Services
College of Ripon and York
St John
York

Nursing Situations 31 minutes
Nine nurse-patient situations presented in order to develop skills in observing and analysing non-verbal communication and to examine different intervention strategies.

Available from:
Didactic Films Ltd
Gatwick House
Horley
Surrey
RH6 9SU
02934 5353

Teaching packs

Teaching Effective Communication in Nursing (Trent Nurse Education Development Project, 1983)
Five-part development of awareness of communication in relation to patient care. Includes exercises, handouts and slides demonstrating non-verbal behaviour.

Available from:
Regional Public Relations Office
Trent Regional Health Authority
Fulwood House
Old Fulwood Road
Sheffield
S10 3TH
0742 306511

Working With Groups (Trainers' Pack)
Handbook from TACADE, Furness House, Trafford Road, Salford M5 2XJ,
061-848-0351. (Introduction to leading groups. Accompanying video available
from Concord Film Council — see above.)

Miscellaneous publications

D. Brandes, *The Gamesters' Handbook II*, Hutchinson, London, 1984.
Structured games and simulations.

J. Jongeward and M. James, *Winning Ways in Health Care: Transactional
Analysis for Effective Communication*, Addison-Wesley, Reading, Mass., 1981.
Exercises in transactional analysis.

J. W. Pfeiffer and J.E. Jones (Eds.) *Handbook of Human Relations Training*,
University Associates, San Diego. Available from People at Work, 159
Chesterfield Road North, Mansfield, Nottingham NG19 7JD. Structured
exercises covering many different aspects of human-relations' training.
Includes mini-lectures covering theoretical material.

P. Priestley and J. Mcguire, *Learning to Help: Basic Skills Exercises*,
Tavistock Publications, London, 1983. Exercises, including interviewing,
counselling, group leading, values and attitudes.

E. Smith, *Choose Happiness and Begin to Take Control of Your Life*, Gateway
Books, London, 1984. Development of awareness of self in our contemporary
environment.

INDEX OF EXERCISES

INDEX